STOP!

IT'S NOT TOO LATE:

Adding Years to Your Life and Life to Your Years Using the BMS Ecosystem

2nd Edition

By

Dr. Harris E. Phillip

Dedication

To my children, Brandon, Kyle, Hillery, and Chantel, whose lives I have tried to steer with the principles contained in this book.

In memory of my loving and caring parents, Burnham, and Blanche Phillip, who doubtlessly sowed the seeds that germinated and blossomed into who I am today.

Table of Contents

Introduction

"Not life, but good life is to be chiefly valued." - Socrates

Have you reached a point on your journey where you feel your life is at a standstill? Perhaps you feel you've reached some sort of peak and that there is nowhere left to go but down. It is not too late to start living a fuller, more productive, and vibrant life! It is not too late to add years to your life and, in turn, to be having such a great time that you will add life to your years. How can you achieve this, and why is it such a secret?

Humans are a triune. We are more complex than just our physical bodies. We are made of three distinct components: Body, Mind, and Spirit. Each component has its own unique characteristics, and all three together create a functioning unit: a human being! Each component (body, mind, and spirit) must be looked after individually to ensure productive and enjoyable years are added to your lives. You can view how to care for each component from the perspective of how you nourish it, what environment you surround it with, and what you allow to impact it.

That is what the **BMS model** is all about. I want to take you through each component and empower you with the appreciation of the value of nourishing yourself appropriately, the environment in which you are nourishing yourself, and finally, bring awareness to what you are allowing to impact you.

You will truly be awarded the tools necessary to integrate all three components of yourself and come to fully understand that through appropriate care, you will add years to your life and life to your years! In the words of Albert Einstein: "Nothing happens until something moves." It is not too late to make something happen, so please make these necessary changes for yourself, so you can start moving and reaping the rewards. Let's dive in!

Foreword

Dear reader…

Do you feel that you try to take care of yourself the best way you know how but always feel that you fall short of your desired energy levels?

Have you ever wondered what the secret to a life full of energy is? Perhaps, you feel that something is missing, or you are constantly struggling to find a sense of balance!

We all want to live a long and healthy life. But what good is a long life if it is not filled with the energy you need to make it your *best* life? Dr. Harris Phillip has not only been practicing medicine for more than 30 years but has also been fascinated by how to create not only a long life but also a vibrant life. This is his life's passion, and he is ready to share it with the world.

He has developed a clear pathway to finding balance and wants this information to now be yours. Not only does his clear observations and reflections make it doable, but it is accessible to every one of us no matter where we are in life. Dr. Phillip takes the idea of our body, mind, and spirit and breaks them down into clear and manageable components of our Self. He will guide you on how to nurture not only each component from the inside out but also the outside in.

If you find this book in your hand, it may be a sign from the Universe that you are ready to live the life of which you always dreamed. It is never too late to make changes and delve deeper into the relationship of your body, mind, and spirit. Let Dr. Phillip remind you that all the tools you need are within arm's reach, and you can reap the benefits of reviving your body, mind, and spirit.

Loral Langemeier,

The Millionaire Maker

Section 1: The Body

"The body politic, as well as the human body, begins to die as soon as it is born, and carries itself the causes of destruction." - Jean-Jacques Rousseau

Your physical body is one part of the very complex structure that makes up the human being. The approach to our revival tends to focus heavily on just the body and not so much on the other equally important components of the triune – the mind and spirit. We will cover those later in the book. I want to focus initially on the physical body. As the American psychologist Abraham Maslow contends, we need to first address our physiological needs before our other needs are met. Maslow was able to structure human needs into a pyramid. He believed that our basic physiological needs form the base of the pyramid, and these needs must first be met before other needs are fulfilled.

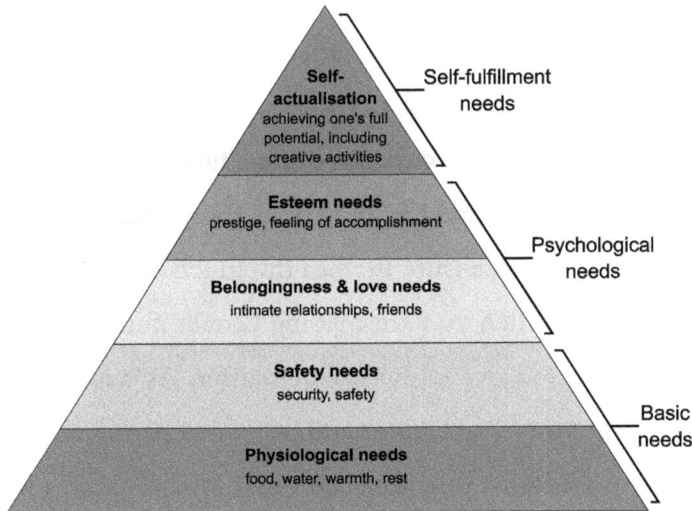

Maslow's Hierarchy of Needs pyramid:

- **Self-actualisation** — achieving one's full potential, including creative activities — Self-fulfillment needs
- **Esteem needs** — prestige, feeling of accomplishment — Psychological needs
- **Belongingness & love needs** — intimate relationships, friends — Psychological needs
- **Safety needs** — security, safety — Basic needs
- **Physiological needs** — food, water, warmth, rest — Basic needs

Chapter 1: Nourishing the Body

"I am conscious of the way I live and do things every day that nourish my body. I eat well, I work out, I try to manage stress, I get a good sleep in, and together, that does wonders." – Ella Woodward

The statement "you are what you eat" is particularly true as the way we nourish ourselves can help us to feel rejuvenated and energetic and help us to be in a pleasant mood, as opposed to feeling dull, dry, and low in energy.

Your food is literally your fuel. When you are looking to revive your physical body, starting with an understanding of fueling yourself is essential. This will create the foundation on which all other parts of your physical revival are based (and subsequently, the revival of your mind and spirit). As we further uncover all the aspects of your revival, the interconnectedness will become clear.

The foods we eat are designed to provide our bodies with various nutrients. I want to focus on the three macronutrients that must be a part of every diet: **carbohydrates**, **fats**, and **proteins**. These nutrients, which are obtained from various foods, need to be ingested in specific quantities to ensure the healthy functioning of our bodies. You will find that when you are missing certain nutrients from your diet, your energy and overall health will suffer. As we uncover what those are, I urge you to take notes and begin comparing your diet as it stands to how a healthy, functional diet may look for you. I know for many of you, it will involve changing your eating habits, patterns, and behaviors. But this is the only way to create a strong foundation for adding years to your life and life to your years. Therefore, this is the starting point of your revival.

Macronutrient #1: Carbohydrates

The most abundant sources of carbohydrates in our food are found in sugar, starch, and fiber. It is from here that carbohydrates are further divided into two categories: **simple** carbohydrates and **complex** carbohydrates. Simple carbohydrates are simple sugars. These are usually refined sugars that you find in many prepared foods, such as cereals and drinks. However, they can also naturally occur in fruits and milk products. The simple sugars that are naturally present in foods in their natural or whole state are a healthier option (compared to the refined version) to consume and may also contain other vitamins and minerals.

Complex carbohydrates are also referred to as starches and include grain products. Some are better food choices than others. White flour, white rice, etc., have been processed and have lost much of their nutritional value and fiber, while unrefined grains still contain their vitamins, minerals, and fiber. Therefore, it is easy to see those unrefined grains, such as brown rice and bulgar wheat, are healthier options. Additionally, they are rich in fiber, which facilitates the optimal functioning of the digestive system. Fiber is also filling and makes you feel satiated sooner and fuller longer, thus reducing the possibility of overeating and weight gain, which can lead to modern diseases of obesity and diabetes (to name a few).

When addressing the carbohydrates in your diet, the best options to ensure you are giving yourself the nourishing foundation you need are whole, unrefined grains, fruits, and vegetables. The daily recommendation for fruit and vegetable intake is about 400 grams per day or five servings of 80grams. A piece of fruit the size of a tennis ball or 2 cups of diced fruits would account for your fruit requirement, and 2 to 2-½ cups of vegetables per day is a useful, workable guide. It is advisable to consume your fruit as first food in the morning after a glass of warm water on an empty stomach. Some fruits, such as citrus, may increase acid production. Fiber and fructose in fruits may slow down the digestive system if eaten on an empty stomach. For this reason, guava and oranges should be avoided in the early mornings. It is unwise to consume your fruits after a meal as they may not be properly digested, and the nutrients may not be properly absorbed. It is recommended that at least 30 minutes be allowed to elapse between a meal and your consumption of fruit. The myth that eating fruit at night allows you to add on weight is just that – a myth.

However, if you consume a calorie-rich fruit like a banana every night after you have completed your calorie requirement for the day, you will add a few pounds by the end of the month. Raw vegetables or a salad should not be consumed on an empty stomach. They contain a lot of coarse fiber, which may increase the work burden on an empty stomach and may lead to flatulence and abdominal pains. There are no digestive benefits in eating your vegetables before, during, or after a meal. Instead, vegetables can be eaten anytime, even as a late-night snack.

Macronutrient #2: Fats

Fats are an important part of our diets. Fats are an integral part of your physical makeup, along with muscle, tissues, and blood. It plays specific roles in the body. Having fat on your body is natural and only becomes a problem when certain types of fat are held onto in excess. There are two types of fat that your body produces: brown fat and white fat. Brown fat helps keep the body warm and is stored in numerous tiny fat droplets. Brown fat is either constitutive (you were born with it, usually showing on adults around the neck and shoulders) or it is recruitable, meaning white fat can be converted to brown fat under appropriate conditions such as cooling your body down (e.g., with an ice bath, stepping out in cold weather, or turning the thermostat in your homes down to about 66°F or 19°C.)

When we eat, the excess nourishment is converted into white fat, which is stored around our various organ systems and is referred to as visceral fat. White fat is the more common variety. White fat stores energy in large fat droplets, which accumulate around the body and surround your internal organs or viscera. White fat keeps you warm through the insulation of your internal organs. It is white fat that leads to obesity, and when stored around your midsection, it leads to the development of the metabolic syndrome, which increases the risk of heart disease, diabetes, and stroke.

There are three major classes of fat: Saturated, Unsaturated, and Trans Fat. Fats are composed of two smaller molecules: glycerol and fatty acids. A **saturated fat** is one in which the fatty acids are composed of single bonds. Saturated fats are solids at room temperature. A small portion of saturated fats is acceptable in your diet. It should comprise only 6% of your daily energy source. At this level, saturated fats can improve your good cholesterol level and change dangerous cholesterol into a more benign form. At higher proportions, the reverse is true. It leads to a build-up of bad cholesterol in our bodies with plaque formation and increased risk of cardiovascular disease.

Sources of saturated fat:

- Fatty cuts of red meat
- Fatty cuts of Pork and chicken with chicken skin and lard
- Dairy foods (milk, butter, cheese, sour cream, ice cream
- Coconut oils, palm oil
- Fried foods

Fats can also be **unsaturated**. These are liquids at room temperature and are the healthier, more beneficial variety. These unsaturated fats improve blood cholesterol levels, reduce inflammation, and stabilize heart rhythms. Unsaturated fats generally have a plant-based origin. They include vegetable oils, nuts, and seeds.

Unsaturated fats is further sub-divided into three types:

1. Monounsaturated fats are found in high concentrations in olives, peanut and canola oils, avocados, almonds, hazelnuts, pecans, pumpkin, and sesame seeds.

2. Polyunsaturated fats are found in high concentrations in sunflower, corn, soybean, flaxseed oils, walnuts, flaxseeds, fish, and canola oil.

3. Omega-3 fats are polyunsaturated and are not produced in the body. They are acquired from the diet by eating fish 2-3 times per week. Omega-3 can be obtained from flax seeds, walnuts, canola, and soybean oil.

The higher the blood content of omega-3 fats, the healthier. Omega-3 fats reduce chronic inflammation in our bodies and lower the risk of premature death among older adults. The evidence suggests that if up to 15% of our daily calories come from polyunsaturated fats, the risk of heart disease is lowered. Recently, we have learned that replacing a carbohydrate-rich diet with one rich in unsaturated fats lowers blood pressure, improves lipid levels, and reduces cardiovascular risk. Coconut oil is particularly rich in saturated fat, containing a larger proportion of saturated fat than a fatty bit of beef. However, coconut oil tends to increase good cholesterol, and therefore, it is a saturated fat with a difference.

Trans Fats are created through an industrial process (i.e., they are not naturally occurring). Hydrogen is added to vegetable oil, which then causes the oil to become solid at room temperature, hence the name "partially hydrogenated oil."

Sources of trans fats include:

- Baked goods such as cakes, cookies, and pies.

- Shortening.

- Microwave popcorn.

- Frozen pizza.

- Refrigerated dough, such as biscuits and rolls.

- Fried foods, including French fries, doughnuts, and fried chicken.

- Non-Dairy coffee creamer.

- Stick margarine.

The reason many restaurants will prefer to use this kind of oil for frying is because of its longer shelf life, so the oil does not have to be changed as often. Unfortunately, trans fats are the worst kinds of fats you can consume. Trans Fats have been shown to raise your bad cholesterol levels while lowering your good cholesterol levels. A diet heavy in trans fats can lead to a higher risk of heart disease, which is the leading cause of death in adults. To keep your body in good health and on a path of revival, be mindful of your consumption of fast food and fried foods and the trans fats that you will be ingesting. Consuming trans fats is a sure ticket to poor health on many levels!

Macronutrient #3: Proteins

Proteins are the third essential macronutrient you require to nourish your physical body. Proteins are made up of building blocks called amino acids that are essential components to all living things. There are three types of proteins based on their function, each playing a specific role in your body. I want to highlight just a few of these features.

Fibrous proteins include keratin and collagen and form part of the connective tissues in the body, such as tendons, bones, and muscles. Therefore, they are necessary for facilitating support and movement. **Globular proteins** may function as enzymes, hormones, transport molecules, and even part of the body's defense system. These types of proteins are integrally involved in the normal functioning of our bodies. The third major type of protein is **membrane proteins**. These are in the actual cell membrane and perform a variety of functions. For example, these proteins may help transport substances across the cell membranes or serve as receptors on which substances can bind and bring about changes within the cell. This is just a glimpse of all the functions of proteins, and as you can see, it goes far beyond just building muscle!

There is a vast array of foods that function as protein sources that are available to us, including:

- lean meat, poultry, fish

- eggs

- dairy products (such as cottage cheese and yogurt)

- seeds and nuts

- beans, legumes (lentils), and soya products

It is recommended that about 12-20% of your daily calories come from protein. Your body stores excess protein as fat. Excess amino acids are transported in the bloodstream to the liver, where they can be used to create new proteins.

Beyond the essential *macro*nutrients of carbohydrates, fat, and protein, your body also requires an array of *micro*nutrients. These include dietary fiber, minerals, vitamins, and water. Every nutrient plays its own specific role when it comes to bringing more vitality to your physical body. Understanding the macronutrients and how they are part of your diet is the essential starting point to reviving your body. When the carbs, fats, and proteins are appropriately balanced in your diet, you will feel more energized, and you will begin to function at a higher level physically. 20-35 % of your total daily calories should come from fat; this means eating 50 to 80 grams of fat per day. On the other hand, carbohydrates should comprise 45-65% of your total daily calories, and 10-30 percent of your daily calories should be made up of proteins. Of course, you can imagine that when that happens, you will begin feeling more vitality.

Reflection:

Am I aware of what I eat, or do I just eat whatever, whenever? How does it make me feel?

Do I eat a good balance of complex carbs to simple carbs?

Do I eat enough healthy fats?

What are the primary sources of protein in my diet?

_____

_____

_____

_____

_____

_____

In the next chapter, I want to give you a snapshot of the basic dietary patterns we follow (omnivore, vegetarian, and vegan) and examine the benefits of them all, so you can begin reflecting on which diet pattern may suit you best. Again, meeting your physiological needs first will set you up for success overall when looking to revive yourself.

Chapter 2: Source of Food

"Want to learn to eat a lot? Here it is eat a little. That way you will be around long enough to eat a lot." – Tony Robbins

Human beings are described as **omnivores** – in that they consume both plant and animal products. This is compared to **carnivores**, whose main sources of nourishment are animal products, and **herbivores**, whose main sources of nourishment are plant-based products. I am sure many of you are asking and wondering which is the best choice when thinking about how to revive your physical body. Let us examine both: a diet that is more animal product-based and one that is more plant-based. There are certainly benefits to each, but the question remains. Which is healthier overall?

I find it fascinating that biblical scholars have rushed to suggest that humans were never to eat animals but were permitted by God because of the lack of vegetation after the great flood in the story of Noah. (These examples are in the book of Genesis.) Other stories found in the bible also show reduced the life span of men, generation after generation, thus further presenting an observation of the human life span, shortening with the introduction of animal-based products to his diet. In today's modern world, which diet is healthier? As we explore these diets, keep in mind we are trying to create a solid and vibrant foundation on which to build.

Carnivore Diet

Supporters of an animal product-based diet believe that meat should be an integral part of your diet because it is filled with nutrients. It is a source of complete high-quality protein, iron, and vitamin B12. Consequently, there are a variety of factors that suggest that meat products in our diet are highly beneficial. Studies have shown that a high protein diet, which includes ingesting meat, can increase your metabolism, reduce hunger, and make you feel fuller longer. (Of course, this can then be associated with weight loss.) Additionally, eating a diet high in animal protein may also help you retain muscle mass, strengthen bones, and help maintain ideal levels of iron in your body. Many people agree that the main benefit of including meat in our diet is that it provides a readily available source of protein, contains all essential amino acids, and further helps build muscle mass.

A snapshot of benefits of having meat in your diet include:

- strengthen bones and aid iron absorption.

- a source of complete amino acids, thus helping build muscle mass.

- strengthen your immune system through the production of antibodies. It contains a full spectrum of micronutrients and vitamins that can promote a healthier state of being.

Having a diet that includes meat products has the potential to contribute to your health. Why is it that there has been a steady decline

17

in the longevity of human beings since meat was introduced into our diets?

In multiple studies by Oxford University, it has been reported that there was an 11% reduced risk of cancer among vegetarians and a 19% reduced risk of cancer among vegans. If we are focusing on adding years to our life and life to our years, would it not then be true to say that a plant-based diet may be the better choice? Could a diet that includes meat products be a contributing factor to illnesses that significantly affect the general population? Since we started consuming meat regularly, there has been a clear increase in heart disease, cancers, strokes, diabetes, obesity, elevated cholesterol levels, acne, and, for men specifically, erectile dysfunction that affects our health year after year – thereby causing a reduction in our overall health and life span.

Let us now explore the virtues of a plant-based diet and all it may offer. It is crucial to be familiar with both diet types when wanting to revive your body so that you may make the most informed decisions for yourself.

The Types of Plant-Based Diets

There are a variety of plant-based diets, and how we distinguish them all depends on their contents.

Lacto Ovo Vegetarian Diet: is one of the most popular plant-based diets. As indicated, no meat (beef, pork, poultry, fish, etc.) is consumed in this diet. Dairy products such as cheese and yogurt are allowed, as well as eggs.

Ovo Vegetarian Diet: Again, excludes all meats and dairy products. Only eggs are ingested in addition to plant-based dishes.

Pescetarian Diet: In this diet, there is no dairy, or eggs consumed along with beef, chicken, and poultry. Only fish and plant-based dishes are consumed.

Vegan Diet: Rising in popularity, a vegan diet excludes all animal-based products in any form. Plant-based dishes are the only foods consumed in this diet.

The Virtues of a Vegetarian Diet

Now presented with the diverse types of vegetarian diets, you are probably wondering which one is the healthiest option for your body. What should you include in your diet, and which foods should you most definitely think of excluding in the long term? Internationally, the vegetarian diet is praised for its health benefits, including lower incidences of heart disease, cancer, and type 2 diabetes. Let us examine a few key elements of a vegetarian diet that can boost your health overall!

Inflammation

An increased number of studies have indicated an association between degenerative diseases and chronic inflammation. Where does this inflammation in the body come from, and how can it be managed? Firstly, inflammation is a naturally occurring process in the body, but it is of two types: acute and chronic inflammation. Our tissues can become inflamed when dealing with an injury, and this is a necessary component of the healing process. Short-term (acute) inflammation differs from chronic inflammation. Chronic inflammation is associated with diseases such as cancers, arterial plaque formation, heart attacks, strokes, diabetes, and autoimmune diseases such as type 1 diabetes and systemic lupus erythematosus (SLE). Chronic inflammation is triggered by free radicals. Free radicals are high-energy particles derived from essential metabolic processes in the human body. They can cause significant disruption to physiological processes. This type of inflammation is seen in diets laden with animal products.

When your body is injured, it will naturally react with inflammation to heal itself. This type of inflammation, acute inflammation, which occurs, for example, after a bruise or a cut, is a healthy natural process.

Studies have shown that eating meat, cheese, and highly processed foods is associated with elevated levels of chronic inflammation in our bodies. This type of inflammation, chronic inflammation, is a dangerous type of inflammation that is associated with chronic diseases. Therefore, it makes good sense to have a plant-based diet rich in fruits and vegetables to stave off the chronic inflammation in your body and give yourself the best opportunity to ward off chronic conditions and diseases.

Microbiome

Trillions of microorganisms live in our body that are collectively known as the microbiome. These microorganisms, while you cannot see them, are crucial to our overall health. They help in the digestion of our foods, produce essential nutrients, contribute to our immune systems, keep our gut tissues healthy, and help to protect against cancer. They also reduce the risk of obesity, diabetes, vascular disease, autoimmune disease, inflammatory bowel disease, and liver disease.

What feeds these healthy microorganisms and bacteria is the fiber found in a variety of fruits and vegetables. When you eat plant-based meals, it promotes the growth of this gut-friendly bacteria. On the other hand, consuming meals high in dairy, eggs, and meat products will help with the growth of disease-promoting bacteria. This negative type of bacteria can lead to diseases such as those listed above. Specifically, is the increased production of Trimethylamine N-oxide (TMAO) found in the bloodstream after consuming animal products. Breaking it down further, consuming the chemicals choline and carnitine, which is found in meats, poultry, eggs, seafood, and dairy, causes the gut bacteria to make Trimethylamine (TMA), which is converted in the liver to Trimethylamine N-oxide (TMAO). It is alarming to note that studies have shown that people with elevated levels of TMAO in their blood have more than twice the risk of a heart attack, stroke, and serious cardiovascular problems compared with people who have lower levels. High TMAO in the blood will lead to chronic kidney disease, increased risk of Type 2 diabetes, and worsening levels of cholesterol plaque in our vascular system (leading to a higher risk of heart disease and stroke).

It is not hard to draw conclusions then, is it?... When you

consume a plant-based diet, you will make little to no TMAO because of your healthier gut microbiome. The benefit of a plant-based diet is quick, as it takes only a few days for the gut's bacterial pattern to change. How exciting to know that making a few changes today can lead to considerable improvements in your gut health and influence your overall health!

The Best Diet for Revival

I'm sure it is now becoming clear that a diet based solely on plants is optimal for your health! This would be what we earlier referred to as a **vegan diet**. Vegan diets are abundant in vitamins B1, C, and E, as well as folic acid, magnesium, and iron. As we now know, an additional benefit is that this diet is low in cholesterol and saturated fats. Cutting out so many foods that you usually consume may make you concerned about any deficiencies in nutrients or vitamins. The concern when going vegan is an increased risk of vitamin B12 deficiency, but it can be easily remedied through the consumption of fortified plant-based food or a straight-up vitamin B12 supplement. (The recommended daily dietary allowance for Vitamin B12 is only 1.8 micrograms for children and adults, 2.4 micrograms for pregnant women, and 2.8 micrograms for breastfeeding women.) Be mindful as well that there are several factors that can affect the absorption of vitamin B12, such as age, antacids, and the drug metformin (commonly used to treat type 2 diabetes).

There are many resources out there that can lead you to a healthy and balanced vegan diet. When using vegan diets, you will not only reap all the benefits we have been discussing but also increase your intake of beneficial antioxidants. Antioxidants optimize how your cells repair damaged DNA and can slow down the ageing process of our cells, which can lead to a more dynamic and longer life!

I do want to briefly touch upon the *quality* of the foods you choose for your diet, as well. To fulfill the world population's demand for food, genetically modified organisms (GMOs) were developed to help increase the yields of crops. However, studies now show that GMO-exposed foods can lead to a multitude of health complications, such as hepatic, pancreatic, renal, and reproductive harmful effects. Knowing this now, I highly recommend that you choose to consume non-GMO foods as much as possible. Another excellent choice is choosing whole foods or foods that are as close to their original state as possible. Even if foods are labeled vegan, they can be highly processed and can aggravate your health. Be mindful and remember, you are what you eat.

The Challenge of Converting to a Vegan Diet: My Personal Experience

I recognize that it is easier said than done. Truly, after eating meat products all your life and now recognizing the virtues of a vegan diet, making a decision to optimize your health so that you may enjoy not only a longer and healthier life, but a more vivacious life is not easy.

For me, I grew up observing the preparation of meat dishes, smelling the enticing aroma of such dishes being prepared, and enjoying the prepared dishes, often craving more, but as I started learning more and more of the virtues of veganism, it became apparent to me that I had to make a change if I wanted to add years to my life and life to my years.

The transition was not easy, with starts and stops along the way. Then I tried through the adage that by the yard, it is hard, but by the inch, everything is a cinch. I dropped red meats from my diet, only using chicken and fish dishes with the occasional relapse of the enjoyment of ox-tail dishes. During the process, I had the opportunity to have a doppler scan on my common carotid arteries, which carries blood to the head, neck, and face.

The results were not pretty, with arterial plaques seen in both arteries, thereby informing me of the risks of having a stroke. When I questioned how the process could be slowed or reversed, the answer was simple: change to a vegan diet. So willing or not, this was a major light bulb moment.

Was I prepared to keep doing what I had always done, but marching slowly to a disabled life, or maybe worse? Was it time to sacrifice the toxins of my meat-eating life and claim an opportunity to feed myself the healthier option of a vegan diet and give myself the foundation for adding years to my life and life to my years? My father, a meat eater, died at age 81, and his mother, a vegan, died at age 115. For me, there was no doubt in my choice since my focus was on the addition of years to my life and life to my years.

I started preparing my own meals, which were bulgur wheat

and lentils. Initially, the taste was repulsive, but with experience and a few tweaks, it became an enjoyable dish. My salads were made with raw cabbage. These were grated, and to add to the attractiveness of the dish, I combined the grated green cabbage with the purple, maroon ones and doused the grated cabbages with colorless apple cider vinegar. I enjoyed this for a while and gradually learned to prepare other dishes. If there is a need for milk in my drinks, I use almond milk. If there is a need for sugar, which is rare, I use stevia.

Since going full-time on my vegan-based meals, the lassitude and need for caffeinated beverages have disappeared. I am experiencing a level of clarity in my thoughts, which reminds me of my twenties. My mood is less fluctuant, and I am always pleasant and friendly. My drive for physical activity has also risen. My bowels are a lot more regular; I have less problem with my weight control, and all in all, I feel more like the self that I consider ideal! I am grateful I am now focusing on a vegan diet, and I love the way it makes me feel.

Hydration: Drinking Enough Water

Where should I begin with all the benefits that staying hydrated can give you? Human beings are composed of at least 65% water. This fact alone should make you understand the importance of drinking enough water throughout the day. You need to make hydration a priority. The reasons we need water and how it affects our body are extensive! I will touch on several key points to get you motivated.

Firstly, you are asking yourself how much water you need to drink to be properly hydrated on any regular day. Health professionals suggest adults should aim for a *minimum* of 2 litres (approx 68 oz) a day. To make it easy to remember, just follow the 8 x 8 principle: have an 8oz glass of water 8 times a day. If you have trouble keeping track of how much water you have consumed throughout the day, I recommend that you drink all your water out of one water bottle throughout the day. Know how many full bottles you need to drink by the end of the day to receive your minimum hydration and keep track of how many times you fill your bottle. (An easy hydration hack!)

The body's response to being dehydrated varies in symptoms and severity. When you are inadequately hydrated, there can be an imbalance in your blood sugar levels, and you may experience headaches or even a change in your mood. Other symptoms may manifest as fatigue, mental slowness, irritability, and a rise in body temperature. When examining all your physiological processes and aspects of physical health there really is nothing for which you do not need an adequate amount of water.

Externally, hydration gives your skin a healthy glow and can reduce the appearance of wrinkles. Water lubricates joints and helps with the delivery of oxygen to our tissues. It also helps in the production of mucus, saliva, and digestive juices. Did you know that water helps in cushioning your brain and spinal cord as well as other sensitive body structures? Hydration keeps these precious organs healthy and free from traumatic physical damage. Water is essential to perspire (your sweat is 90% water!), which not only helps regulate body temperature (even when you are not working out) but also aids in excreting toxins from the body.

One point that is not touched upon but which I feel may be of interest is the correlation between hydration and managing your weight. Water can function as an appetite suppressant and seems to allow our bodies to use up more calories in our resting state. In some animal studies, water was shown to have a fat-burning capacity. Therefore, if you are trying to manage your weight, staying adequately hydrated has an important part to play in your efforts.

Can you consume too much water? The answer is *yes*! However, for the average, healthy person, this would be extremely hard to do. Your kidneys are responsible for eliminating water from your body and can eliminate 0.8 to 1L of fluid every hour. Therefore, you may run into problems when you drink *more* than a litre of water every hour. Excessive water in our system causes a diluted amount of sodium in our body, which can then lead to an excess of fluid being absorbed into our cells and resulting in swelling. Obviously, taking the body out of this homeostasis (balanced) state can be harmful to your health on many levels. Sticking to the ideal of 2L/day will not only make you feel better physically, but it also leads to positive outcomes for your mind and spirit. You will *feel* better by drinking more water! What an inexpensive and quick solution for many things that may be ailing you.

Reflection:

What kind of diet am I currently eating?

Why would I consider switching to a plant-based diet?

Are there any benefits to me in switching to a plant-based diet?

What will it take for me to switch to a plant-based diet?

Am I willing to switch to a plant-based or vegan diet?

What are my favorite fruits and vegetables?

How much water do I drink in a day on average?

Have I noticed a correlation between what I eat and how I feel physically (Does the food I eat contribute to aches I feel or digestive issues, etc.?)

_____

_____

_____

_____

_____

_____

_____

_____

_____

_____

Of course, I am going to encourage you to grab a glass of water and continue reading on, while we continue exploring how we can elevate the health of our physical body to create a solid foundation for your revival. Let us start looking at elements around you that can have a great impact, specifically air and sunlight.

Chapter 3: The Environment We Live In

"Although our bodies are bounded with skin, and we can differentiate between outside and inside, they cannot exist except in a certain kind of natural environment." – Alan Watts

To say that we do not live in a vacuum is undoubtedly stating the obvious! As we go about our "day-to-day" activities, there is no denying that the environment around us deeply impacts our physical bodies, both positively and negatively. In an effort to stay in line with our goal of adding years to your life and life to your years, it is worth taking some time to investigate some major aspects of your environment, reflect on how they are affecting you now, and how you can make some changes in order to harness the most positive aspects of both **air** and **sunlight** that surrounds you.

Air

When you think of your relationship with air, you may think solely of the oxygen that we need to breathe. However, oxygen only composes about 21% of the volume of air surrounding us. The air around us is a blanket that acts as a sort of environmental shield for our bodies. It maintains temperature by trapping heat from the sun (this regulated temperature is vital for our bodies), and it protects our bodies from the harmful effects of ultraviolet radiation from the sun.

The ozone layer, a part of the earth's atmosphere, is integrally involved in shielding us from the harmful effects of ultraviolet radiation. This complex process involves absorbing the bulk of ultraviolet radiation from the sun. Air also acts as a medium through which the carbon dioxide we exhale is absorbed by plants to produce food through photosynthesis. Plants in the process give off oxygen, which we use for our own nourishment through respiration.

When you have access to clean air, it can help improve your blood pressure and heart rate and facilitate digestion. It can strengthen your immune system and help clear your lungs. Exposure to fresh air leads to an improvement in mood, energy levels, and a sharper mind. Breathing is an automatic phenomenon; putting focus on the quality of air we breathe is helpful.

The bottom line is we require clean air to live optimally! For those of us who live in more urban areas where the air quality may not be stellar. Being mindful to take a walk in the early morning hours when the air quality is better is ideal. If you live in a more rural setting where there is less pollution, going outside at a minimum once a day, preferably in the morning, for a 30-minute walk can be rewarding. When outside during your walks, focus on your breathing and perhaps take deeper breaths than usual. This will aid in the fresh air really entering deep into your lungs and helping deliver all its benefits to your body. Having a daily dose of clean air, while such a simple act, will make a significant impact on your revival!

Global warming and climate change are having a deleterious effect on our life, including our health and the air we breathe. Global warming is blamed for the buildup of greenhouse gases (such as carbon dioxide and methane) in the atmosphere, causing ambient temperatures to rise. Using fossil fuels for travel and the farming of animals are major contributors to this environmental damage. Combined with rapid deforestation and fewer trees to absorb carbon dioxide and produce oxygen. It is a recipe for ill health for us overall. If the temperature of ambient air on the planet continues to rise, it will make living conditions on Earth that much harsher and may eventually render the planet uninhabitable. If we do not come together (citizens and leaders alike) to take full responsibility for this issue, our health and the well-being of future generations cannot be guaranteed.

I am sure you have read about how you can be effective in addressing the issue of global warming. One definitive way of acting and making a change on a personal level is choosing to have a plant-based diet. Not only is it beneficial for your body, as we discussed in the previous chapter, but it is also beneficial for the environment!

You may not be aware, but creating less of a demand for animal products affect the health of our planet. Animal farming is one of the greatest contributors to global warming. For example, take the production of beef and its extreme production of methane gas (which is eighty times more powerful in causing environmental destruction than carbon dioxide over a 20-year period). Could you imagine the positive long-term atmospheric changes if people were to reduce the amount of beef and other animal products they consume or choose to stop eating animal-based products altogether? Choosing a plant-based diet is really a win-win situation when you look at it through this lens.

Good for you and good for the planet!

Sometimes, you may not be able to see or feel the direct effects of what is contaminating the air around you. Great technological advances are certainly improving our lives in multiple ways by allowing great ease of communication, helping us to stay connected, and creating business opportunities. However, with the move to more online-based communication and the demand for it to be faster every year comes an increase in various sources of electromagnetic radiation. This type of air pollution is one we cannot see or initially feel, but it most certainly is there, present beyond our immediate control. We trust scientific communities and governments to safeguard our interests and our health when it comes to this specific element in our environment. However, now that you know electromagnetic radiation is adversely affecting your environment and can affect your well-being, it is empowering as you can now advocate for your own health and safety.

Living in polluted cities and towns is part of living in this modern era. We cannot escape it, and it is something we must learn to navigate. Therefore, it is of utter importance that you remember each breath you take can impact your health. Getting out in the early morning for some fresh air or taking steps to reduce the electromagnetic pollution in your home (i.e., turning off electronics when not in use and/or reducing use altogether) is imperative for reviving your body. Acting for your health empowers you. Empowering yourself is part of reviving yourself.

Sunlight

Your relationship to sunlight is an essential pillar in leading a healthy and active life. It is a natural part of our surroundings and environment, which we too often take for granted. One of the most popular benefits of exposing yourself to sunlight is an increase in your body's production of vitamin D. Our body produces Vitamin D when exposed to the sun! Vitamin D is vital in combating chronic inflammation. It lowers blood pressure, improves brain function, and helps improve your mood. It helps strengthen bones and teeth as well. As you can see, Vitamin D is vital to being healthy. It is no wonder that when you live in the northern hemisphere, it is recommended that you take a vitamin D supplement during the winter months when you are exposed to much less sunlight. You will agree that during the winter months, there is much less sunlight, and the colder temperatures keep you indoors, thereby further robbing you of exposure to sunlight and daylight.

While we are talking about winter months with less sunlight, it is important to touch upon Seasonal Affective Disorder (SAD). SAD is a mood disorder where people express depressive symptoms during the winter months. There is a direct correlation between increased cases of SAD and less sunlight. Sunlight produces serotonin (the "feel good hormone") in the body. It is no wonder that a widely accepted treatment for SAD is light therapy. Light therapy is the exposure to an artificial light source that is not a source of UV light. The light enters through the eye and, in a sense, tricks the brain. The production of serotonin is triggered by light entering the eye, so even if you are not exposed to the sun itself, having a light box handy on your desk or at home can ensure that serotonin is produced, even without a daily dose of sun or daylight. (Light boxes are readily available for purchase online or at wellness stores.) Light therapy may prove to be an inexpensive way to naturally boost your mood, and, therefore, your overall wellness. I urge you to try it!

For your well-being, I must mention that there are hazards to excessive exposure to the sun. Sun exposure can lead to skin damage, such as sunburn, premature skin ageing, and even cancer. (Frighteningly, 90% of skin cancers are caused by exposure to the sun.) Avoiding direct sunlight, especially in the afternoon when the sun's ultraviolet light is most potent, is best. I am not saying to totally avoid the sun as that is also detrimental to your health. I just ask you to remain mindful as to what time of day you are going to expose yourself to the sun and for how long. At all other times, be mindful to stay covered and use appropriate sunscreen.

Reflection:

How often do I get out in the morning for fresh air?

How often do I go outside for some sunlight?

Do I ever feel like I have a low mood in the winter months?

Does your mood in the winter months differ from the summer months?

_____

_____

_____

_____

_____

_____

_____

I hope that you are feeling even more inspired now to go outside for fresh air and sunlight and consider a plant-based diet. In our modern lives that revolve around work and screen time, it is easy to forget about how such simple factors like clean air and a daily dose of sunlight are necessary to truly live our best life. There are more critical aspects to the foundation one must create to gain vitality and add years to your life and life to your years. The final building blocks I want to discuss are being physically active, the importance of rest, and the necessity of temperance. It is always about keeping things in balance.

Chapter 4: Factors That Impact Your Body

"Nothing happens until something moves." – Albert Einstein

The final key when you are reviving your body is to look at things you have control over that impact your physical self. I want us to examine exercise, rest, and the practice of temperance. These are the final pieces when creating that solid foundation, you need to continue your journey of adding more years to your life and life to your years. Let us first discuss the importance of getting your heart pumping with physical exercise!

Benefits of Physical Exercise

Our bodies love to move! We are expected to move. It is not a coincidence that when we move our bodies endorphins (the "feel good chemicals") are released, helping reduce stress and boost our mood. Our bodies will reward us for exercising. However, the key is to start moving.

In our modern lives, we live amazingly comfortable lives. Technology is making it easier to work and communicate. It is as if everything is at our fingertips. However, with these advances have also come a more sedentary lifestyle. We are spending an unprecedented amount of time in front of screens, either working or entertaining ourselves. Being inactive for extended periods of time has resulted in lifestyle-related diseases such as obesity, diabetes, and high blood pressure. If you think about it, even just simply walking may be excluded from your daily activities depending on where you live and where you work. People simply drive around. So, think of it like this: you drive from home (where you spend a lot of time in front of your TV or computer watching shows or playing games) to work, where you likely spend a lot of your time in front of a screen (depending on your job of course). This cycle is cutting out the physical activity we require to feel good and boost our general health.

Physical activity also sets you up for success if you are looking to lose weight. Maintaining a healthy weight is part of your revival. Sometimes, the missing piece of the puzzle for those on a weight loss journey is not getting enough exercise. It is simply not enough to change your diet. When physical activity becomes part of your lifestyle, your efforts, and any weight loss you experience will help to maintain the weight loss over the months and years. Your metabolism changes as you age, and being physically active helps boost your metabolism and, therefore, maintain your weight well into your golden years.

Physical exercise is not only necessary for your health, but also vital. It is a practice necessary to add years to your life and life to years. Let us examine the main types of physical exercise and their benefits. If you do not already have an exercise regime, I want to offer you a starting point. If exercise is already part of your life, you find yourself always enjoying cardio-based exercise as opposed to resistance training. I want to give you insight into the importance of keeping both aerobic and strength training in balance.

Types of Exercise and the Importance of Intensity

Since we are focusing on ensuring you add years to your life and life to your years, I would suggest we examine basic aerobic and strength training exercises. Both categories can be broken down further into many subgenres, but let's start with an overview so that you may feel inspired. I am especially looking to those of you who may not have a regular exercise routine. A weekly exercise routine is necessary for reviving your body; it is attainable, and it can be fun!

When looking at your weekly aerobic needs, you may already be contributing to them without even realizing it. About 150 minutes of *brisk* walking, swimming, biking, gardening, or even weekly lawn-mowing is all it takes to start a routine. Alternatively, if your fitness level is already in a good spot, you may want to engage in activities that are more rigorous and challenging (after consulting with your doctor first to ensure you are approaching a new routine safely).

This can look like aerobic dancing or running for 75 min/week. If you have the time and motivation, or if you feel you would like a further challenge, incorporating three hundred minutes (5 hours) per week will really make a difference in how you feel in your body. Do not do yourself a disservice by negating this amount of aerobic exercise. You can easily do 5 hours a week by doing a bit every day and starting new daily healthy exercise habits. Over the course of a week, you will see that every effort can really add up!

Now, let us not forget about the strength training. Strengthening all your major muscle groups is ideally done for a minimum of 2x/week. You can use free weights or weight machines, but if those are not available to you, simply engage in activities with your own weight resistance such as using a pull-up bar or rock climbing. Heavy gardening may even be appropriate here. Just remember it can be as simple as using your own weight as resistance, whatever that may look like. (If you need suggestions, there are a plethora of resources online.)

The effectiveness of both aerobic exercise and strength training comes down to your intensity level when moving. There is quite a difference between going for a leisurely walk and going for a brisk walk when it comes to affecting your health. Your activity level should be at a moderate or vigorous level of intensity. However, what this feels like is based solely on the individual, as everyone is at various levels of physical fitness. What may be a challenging routine for one person may feel easy to the next. An effective way to start gauging this is by assessing your breathing while working out. When you moderately exert yourself, you will break a sweat after about 12 minutes and will feel comfortable having a conversation but have difficulty singing. When participating in more vigorous activity, you will break a sweat after five to seven minutes of your workout, and you will only be able to express yourself in short sentences or a few words, needing to stop and catch your breath more often.

Using these guidelines is a fantastic way to really assess where you are at with your exertion levels. You may also monitor your heart rate, of course, but you will require a heart monitoring system attached to you (ex., a Fitbit or something similar) or have to stop and do calculations on the spot. I like to keep things straightforward and simply just connect with my breathing.

Please keep in mind that you can always *over-exert* yourself. If you find that you are short of breath or are experiencing chest pains, it is usually an indication of working beyond your capacity at the moment. There is a fine line between engaging in vigorous activity and pushing yourself too far. Learn to know where your physical threshold is and build up your stamina and strength step by step over time. This is a lifelong practice, so I urge you to be mindful and stay safe. As you can see, you do not even need a lot, if any, equipment to get in your exercise. All you need is to get out of your own way!

Reflection:

Do I have a physical fitness routine?

What do I tend to lean towards, aerobic activity or strength training?

How can I incorporate more physical fitness activity into my day and week?

How can I make being more physically active a priority?

_____

_____

_____

_____

_____

_____

The Importance of Rest

Rest is essential to our physical well-being and all levels of our revival. We may have been conditioned to attribute the idea of rest to being lazy or trying to avoid work. On the contrary, you require rest to work at your highest potential (be it physically or otherwise). Rest allows for recovery, resuscitation, repair, rebuild, and revival of the physical body and mind. Resting improves cardiovascular health, lowers blood pressure, and reduces stress hormones like cortisol. Your mood, alertness, mental clarity, creativity, and motivation are improved with rest (which, in turn, improves your productivity and quality of life). Vacations reduce the risk of heart disease and increase lifespan.

We work long hours to keep up with our growing workloads, running the risk of burnout in the process as we desperately try to keep up. Vacations become a second thought as we battle stress, illness, and the constant pressure to find time for all our commitments outside work. Rest is an essential part of doing our best work and being more productive at work. According to the Institute for Work and Families, fewer than half of U.S. employees take all their vacation days, and Glassdoor reported that 61% of employees work during vacation. Individuals tend to think of vacation as an indulgence that we cannot afford, but it is a necessary part of doing your best work.

Various authors have indicated the benefits of taking a vacation and have advanced at least eight benefits of taking a vacation:

1. The office is not a place for inspiration, so getting away gives you an opportunity to draw on your creativity.

2. Leaving the office moves you away from your comfort zone, thereby giving you an opportunity for a unique perspective.

3. Your health benefits enormously. One study showed that 82% of small business owners who took a vacation were performing better at work when they returned. As a bonus, about a third of men who took a vacation were less likely to die of heart disease.

4. It allows your brain to get a break from the continued daily grind that the office and that environment present.

5. You may not realize it, but a change of scenery is necessary as it strangely gives new life to your endeavors.

6. It facilitates networking.

7. It allows you to realize that the office can be run without you, thereby facilitating delegating, and minimizing the stress that comes with overworking yourself.

8. It keeps both yourself and your workers happy. It allows them to recognize their importance to the company and will encourage them to do their best work.

Sleep is one of the most important aspects of rest as it allows you to regenerate not only your physical self but your mind and spirit as well. Experts tell us that there are two basic types of sleep. Rapid eye movement sleep and non-rapid eye movement sleep. The non-rapid eye movement sleep is divided into three stages. Stage 1 is the changeover from wakefulness to sleep; stage 2 is the period of light sleep before entering stage 3, which is deep sleep. It is during deep sleep that glucose metabolism in the brain increases, supporting both short and long-term memory and overall learning. It is during deep sleep that the pituitary gland in the brain secretes essential hormones, such as growth hormones, which leads to the growth and development of the body. Deep sleep allows for other benefits, such as energy restoration and cell regeneration. The blood supply to muscles increases. During sleep, tissues and bones get repaired, and the immune system is strengthened.

It is recommended that adults get six to eight hours of sleep each night, no excuses! You must be mindful that you are ensuring you facilitate an uninterrupted, restful sleep each night to feel constantly alert and refreshed. Therefore, it is ideal that you create a solid sleep regime for yourself. This starts by committing to start winding down a minimum of 45 min before you would like to sleep (This varies among individuals, some people need more). Start this time by avoiding any distractions (ex., pets, TV, discussions with partners, anything to do with your phone, etc.) and allowing your mind to begin a process of relaxation. A warm shower or bath can help you to begin to relax for bedtime; so, does a cup of warm almond milk.

Also, ensure your bedroom is at an appropriate temperature for sleep (no cooler than twenty degrees Celsius or 68°F). Be mindful that the absence of light (or very dim light) will trigger the production of the hormone melatonin, which is essential for your sleep/wake cycle. Persons may find calm and gentle music, as well as pink noise, help them to continue to relax and drift off to sleep (personal taste can vary with this, and I suggest you do research as there are many free online resources). Getting serious about cultivating and sticking to your sleep regime will be a game changer in your life.

Beyond sleep, it is also ideal to have one full day of rest a week as well. This allows you to slow down and revive yourself. When you rest by taking a day off from your usual schedule, you will gain increased drive and inspiration for the tasks that lie ahead. For many this is naturally built into your regular calendars with the weekend days. We rarely work all seven days of the week and taking at least one day over the weekend for rest and play is ideal. A day off for rest does not simply imply that you laze about or sleep for that day. Resting can look like changing your focus on that day and engaging with something other than work, be it playing a game, relaxing with friends, or spending quality time with family. It is a rest from your daily chores and, therefore, will serve to re-energize you and provide you with useful mental relaxation.

Cultivating a strong relationship with both exercise and rest is essential. Creating this balance will allow you to sustain a definitive tempo in your days, as opposed to a cycle of burnout and then needing to recover. Your energy will be sustained, and your life will improve dramatically.

Reflection:

How many hours of sleep do I get on average?

Do I have healthy sleep habits?

How do I feel about taking a break or an actual day off to rest

and enjoy myself?

How easy is it to drift off to sleep?

What distractions interfere with my ability to drift off to sleep?

How can I improve the quality of my restful sleep?

How do I take downtime in my life?

_____

_____

_____

_____

_____

_____

_____

_____

_____

_____

Temperance

Everyone deserves to enjoy life to the fullest! "Eat, drink and be merry!" is a common saying. Can you remember the last time you overindulged? Could it be eating too much of your favorite food or having too much to drink? How did it make you feel? When you throw yourself into anything with total abandon, it is more difficult to exercise self-control, and having the ability not to overindulge is essential when encouraging the revival of your body. Exercising temperance is necessary to add years to your life and life to your years. Avoiding excess in all areas of your life is essential for healthy living. Practicing self-control is like anything: the more you practice it, the better you become at it.

If you are at a loss for what temperance may look like, the feeling of temperance is found within. Your body will send you strong signals as to when you are at the line of "enough." It is up to you to learn how to hear and feel these signals. Take, for example, you are eating your absolute favorite meal. You may finish half your plate and feel quite satisfied, but you keep eating anyway because it tastes so good. After you finish eating, instead of feeling just full enough and satisfied, you feel overly full and wish you had stopped when you felt satisfied. Your body knows its limits, and it expects you to listen.

The practice of temperance easily extends into all aspects of one's life. We previously talked about physical activity. This is an area where temperance becomes important as well. If you overexert yourself and you push beyond your own limits, this may result in injury. If you over-exercise you do not give your muscles enough time to recover and repair, which is an essential part of gaining strength and endurance. Exercise regimes have both aerobic and strength training, swinging back and forth between the two in equal measure. It is constantly about balance.

The catholic catechism describes temperance as the moral virtue that moderates the attraction of pleasure and provides balance. Again, it is not about denying yourself pleasure but about developing mastery of your own will so that you may keep your desires within limits. This is not only honorable but makes you feel good. Anything done in excess invariably has an adverse effect on our bodies. It is your responsibility to take temperance into consideration when reviving all parts of yourself. It is a fine balance to find within. But I assure you when you find this balance, you will feel fantastic, and inspired. You will reap all the benefits that temperance has to offer. Your body will reward you with a vibrancy like you have never experienced before and you will continue to feel good throughout your years!

Reflection:

In what areas in your life does balance come easy?

Where do you feel you push too hard and overextend yourself?

Where do you feel you push too little and not meet your own potential?

How can you apply more temperance in your life starting today?

What does temperance look like in your life on a grander scale?

_____

_____

_____

_____

_____

_____

_____

_____

_____

_____

We have finished examining the various aspects of reviving our physical bodies. We discussed the importance of choosing the right foods to fuel yourself and how that may contribute to your world beyond your plate. We touched upon our relationship to sunlight and fresh air. The importance of moving your body was brought to the forefront, as well as the need to rest, and how it is all about creating balance and inviting temperance into your life.

I hope you are feeling inspired to cultivate changes in your relationship with your physical self so that you may live your daily life with vitality and joy. Remember, your body will collaborate *with* you, not against you. It is a matter of developing a strong relationship with it and offering your body what it needs so that it may serve you for years to come!

In part two of this book, we will move on to exploring the next component of the triune: your mind. We will explore and uncover the relationship you have with your mind so that you may nourish it appropriately to cultivate its revival. Of course, this will start with discussing what the mind is! It is not something you can see or feel, but it is an integral part of you, nonetheless. Working on the revival of your mind is the next step to adding years to your life and life to your years.

PART TWO: THE MIND

Have you ever wondered about the impact of your mind on your behavior, character, and your body? In medical school doctors will recall the attempts by our professors to consider some illnesses as psychosomatic illnesses. Simply put this describes the impact of the mind in causing the body to experience ill health. The impact of the mind on our beings is best memorialized by the negro poet Cowper, in his 1788 poem, the Negro's Complaint, in his reflection on the dehumanization of slavery, this Caucasian gentleman was able to keep his chin up in his poem an extract of which went as follows.... *Still in thoughts as free as ever, what are England's rights I ask, me from my delights to sever, me to torture, me to task? Fleecy locks and black complexion cannot forfeit nature's claim; skins may differ, but affection dwells in whites and blacks the same. If I were so tall as to reach the pole or to grasp the ocean at a span, I must be measured by my soul, the mind is the standard of the man.'* Dr Martin Luther King endorsed the role of the mind through his use of bits of Negro poet Cowper writings in his speeches. Other authors and professors have addressed the same concept in diverse ways, for example Professor Roy Meadow postulated the term Munchausen Syndrome by proxy which by extension massages the concept of the power of the mind over the body. It is therefore not farfetched to explore the role of the working of the mind in the evolution of the healthiest and best version of oneself. Muhammad Ali understood the importance of the workings of the mind as embodied in his reflective statement....*"I hated every minute of training, but I said, don't quit. Suffer now and live the rest of your life as a champion."* - Muhammad Ali

We at Philburn Academy will help you to understand this concept and seek to massage your mindset to allow you to evolve into the healthiest version of you, as the proponents of the BMS ecosystem, we realize the critical role played by the mind in the success of this approach. A simple belief about yourself permeates every aspect of your life.

We see the attempt by our fellow men to dull the impact of their minds by exposing themselves to a plethora of mind altering substances, be it alcohol or other harmful drugs, marijuana, cocaine and its various cousins in an attempt to undergo a mental drift away from the effects of a functioning mind, some people may claim this mental drift as an attempt to step away from reality. Surely there is a personality type which is drawn to that type of behavior, yet the substances used, though it eventually affects the body, the primary purpose is for immediacy of the mind alteration that results from the use of these substances.

Would you therefore, as a minimum, appreciate the evidence suggests that our minds play a governing role over our bodies? it provides appropriate guidance which will be immeasurable in our journeys of becoming the healthiest, most active versions of ourselves Our foods consumed take care or is supposed to take care of our physical bodies, but our mind governs our thought process, and the combination creates the image that society chooses to refer to as our personality.

It is based on the impact of this thought process that people differ. We will describe our sporting champion in one light, our successful businessmen in a different light, successful relationships may also be viewed in a different light, and we are even sold tools to allow us to reap successes in certain endeavors, but on closer analysis though the recipe may differ the acquisition of the desired outcome lies in the sandwich of mindset.

Why is it that you feel fear when breaking new ground, or in common parlance getting out of your comfort zone? Yet there are many people moving forward anyways despite this fear? Einstein states the truism that nothing happens until something moves but we introduce a slight alteration to Einstein view to read nothing happens until the mind evolves, usually through the acquisition of new experiences in the school of life. In this section I want to explore the second exponent of the BMS ecosystem. The second step is all about your mind and how you can create changes to continue building yourself in line with adding years to your life and life to your years. Let us first discuss exactly what the mind is in an individual.

Chapter 5: An Introduction to Your Mind

"The trained mind is a rich mind." – Robert Kiyosaki

Inherent in Kiyosaki's statement is that the mind can be trained. Even before our time, humankind grappled with trying to find a reason people differ. Through the ages, various hypotheses have been advanced, among them phrenology, a field of study that looks at the conformation of the skull as an indication of mental faculties and character traits. Others focus on craniology; here, the size and shape of the head is used as a sort of predictor of mental faculties and character traits. The discussion continues and now has evolved into, is it nature (genes) or is it the environment (nurture) that determines who we become? Irrespective of your allegiance, I prefer to think that both contribute and likely in variable amounts. Thus, the final product cannot be fully attributed to nature, nor can it be purely because of the environment. It is the contribution of the environment that Kiyosaki seems to be talking about. I believe Gilbert Gottlieb, the eminent neuroscientist, puts it best: he says, 'not only do genes and environment cooperate as we develop, but the genes require input from the environment to work well.'

It is now emerging that people have the capacity for lifelong learning and brain development. If that is so, then since our genetic endowment does not change – we have the potential for growth with time. The interaction between the fixed genetic endowment and the capacity and willingness for change. Effective learning makes change inevitable, so humankind continues to metamorphosize with time. It is on this basis we believe that the BMS ecosystem can add years to your life and life to your years because of its teachings. Once you understand and implement the concepts, we expect the results to be a longer and more active life. If I may borrow the words of Robert Sternberg, one perceived to be an intelligence expert, he postulates that the major factor in whether people achieve excellence is not prior ability but purposeful engagement. Alfred Binet recognized that those who start out the smartest may not end up the smartest – indicating strongly that training/the environment can effect change in outcome. The mind is, therefore, not a fixed construct.

What is the actual mind? Where does it live, and how does it serve us? What is its relationship to the other components of self (the body and spirit)? The mind is described as the set of cognitive faculties, including consciousness, imagination, perception, thinking, judgment, language, and memory, which are housed in the brain. It allows for imagination, recognition, and appreciation and contributes to feelings and emotions. So again, the brain is the physical mass that is a part of our body systems and houses the mind. Yet the mind exists within its own realm and is intertwined with the physical being as well as the spirit.

How is it that while one person may be willing to step forward and continue to grow as a person, even in the face of fear, another may shrink? What exactly is this unique differentiating character with which some are gifted? We all feel fear when trying something new. It is part of our human experience! There are two types of people. Ones that tend to always be looking back, blaming others, or constantly looking at the negative side of things and the others who think positively. Positive thinking, as Zig Ziglar contends, will let you do everything better than negative thinking will. Albert Einstein advises that we stay away from negative people because they have a problem for every solution. Those who say the glass is half full are positive thinkers and are willing to take a risk and believe that there are always better opportunities for themselves. With some commitment, desire, and application, they strive to move the glass from being half full to full or fuller. What is the driving force in these people? Is it their minds? specifically, their **mindset?** The view one adapts to their life affects the way they live their life. It can determine whether you become the person you want to be and what you accomplish.

If you believe your qualities are fixed, you are burdened by the need to prove it to yourself. For example, if one continues to tell a child that he or she is smart, then it does something to the child's mind, making it difficult to address challenges or failures. Similarly, telling a child that he is foolish will cause the child to accept failure and suboptimal performances as his best result since his condition places a sealing on what he/she is able to achieve. Considering the room for growth afforded by nurture, are we then mere unprocessed material acted upon by nurture? Should we accept that we, at any stage of our lives, are mere foundations on which much can be built? We are of the view that growth is possible in all, but it requires desire and application.

Therefore, it is impossible to predict or know a person's true potential. It is impossible to know the result of years of passion, toil, and training. If you have the passion for having years added to your life and life to your years and you are willing to work at it, with the appropriate training, you will get there and grow into your greatness. The history of humankind is replete with countless stories of folks who were considered just average by their peers and even advised to seek a career in other disciplines, with application, hard work, and training, they exceeded many expectations. Of recent memory is Michael Jordan, the retired USA basketball player, who did not make his high school basketball team. This, he claims, ignited a passion within him, and now, years later, he is considered around the world to be the greatest basketball player of all time.

Examination of your mindset is not a modern concept. Throughout the ages, the inquiry of mindset has been a constant in human study. Repeatedly, there have been writings and reflections on the adverse reactions of people who blame other people or things for not moving forward or why they may not have had more of an opportunity extended to them. One such story that really highlights this for me is the Parable of Talents that we find in the Bible. This is a notable example of someone squandering a great opportunity, with the classic behavior of a negative thinker, finding excuses solely because of their mindset.

The Parable of Talents

In the Parable of Talents, the story is of a rich man who had three servants. Upon departure for a trip, he gives each of his servants a portion of his riches in talents. (Talents here refer to money in the form of seed capital thought to each be worth a modern sum of over a million dollars!) The first servant received five talents, the second received three talents, and the third servant received one talent. The master tells them to care for his money, and the first two servants go forth and use their talents to trade and gain profit. When the master returns, the servants one and two give him back double the talents which they received! He is so impressed that he gives them back a portion of the money, which for his servants is a life-changing gift, no doubt. However, the third servant, fearful of the gift, simply hides/buries the talent and returns it as is to the master upon his return. The master scolds and chides him for not being willing to take advantage of investing and trying to create profit, even with only one talent.

There was no difference between the servants themselves. The only difference was their mindset and how they viewed the gifts given to them. The first two servants saw their glasses as half *full,* **an opportunity,** and went forward with enthusiasm and curiosity to try to fill the glass. The third, however, wasted an opportunity to invest and grow because, to him, the glass was half empty. He then had to do everything that he could to prevent the glass from becoming empty; to him, his safest option was to bury the talent which he received. There was no self-motivation.

Was it because of his mindset that he was unable to invest his talent and so received nothing? Observe people around you. Study people at your work, places of worship, and even people in public spaces. You will begin to clearly see a distinction between the two types of mindsets. In simplest terms, some people will see the glass as half-full, an opportunity to fill the glass, and others will see the glass as half empty, fearful that they may lose the contents of the glass and render it empty, creating difficulty with a granted opportunity.

Let us look at the scenario a bit more closely. Firstly, we are not all given equal opportunities. A single opportunity should be sufficient. We are alive, which is one opportunity, that is all we need. **LIFE is the opportunity we need** to grow into our greatness. The same object being looked at by two different individuals produced different perspectives. The major difference is their mindset and the interpretation of what they see. It is particularly intuitive that one individual sees the glass with a positive outlook. The glass is half full, inherently, suggesting the possibility of filling it up. The other sees the glass as being half empty, empty here being a negative connotation and, by extension, an indication of the mindset. The interpretations suggest one of hope and opportunity whilst the other suggests one of fear and the need for protection. The one of hope and opportunity see the half-full glass with the hope that it can be filled, if the right steps are taken. The other who sees the glass as half empty is paralyzed with fear that the glass is almost empty. It is halfway there, so any action that he undertakes may result in the glass becoming empty. Hence, there is a need to protect it. Hide it or even bury it, if you will, as in the story of the talents above. Therefore, our mindsets go a long way in determining how we interpret what we see, and they also guide our next steps.

Reflection:

Why would a glass being half full motivate?

Why would a glass being half empty discourage?

Are you willing to work with the gifts that you have been given?

Who in your life sees the glass as half full?

Who sees it half empty?

How are you affected by their behavior?

Have you ever blamed someone or something in your life instead of taking ownership or responsibility for it?

_____

_____

_____

_____

_____

_____

_____

_____

_____

_____

_____

_____

The Influences of The Mind

As we mentioned, the brain is the physical mass that is a part of our body system and houses the mind. The mind exists within its own realm and affects our physical being. This is why it is imperative to understand your mind and how it works so that you may work on its revival, as you did with the body. (Never forget the three components of the person are all interconnected!)

The body is a mere vehicle for the carriage of our minds and spirit, so, our bodies are mere vessels that are directed by our minds, and to some degree, our spirit guides the direction of the mind, which gives rise to our personality, beliefs, and traits. Recall that the negro poet Cowper long told us the mind is the standard of the man.

To connect with your mind, you must first fully understand that the truths that you perceive around you first begin with your mind, and our belief system colors it. The world around you is constantly relaying negativity towards you, and it is your mind, conditioned by your spirit, which will decide what you do with it. This starts right from the time you are born with the closest people around you while growing up (your family, teachers, and caretakers) and continues into your adulthood.

Obviously, our family and caretakers thought they were doing an outstanding job of protecting us from ourselves, a role now employed by an aspect of the mind called the ego. The ego is an aspect of our mind that has been formed from your conditioning and habits. This is the protective or rational part of the mind. It restrains us or seeks to restrain us from risky behavior. Based on the workings of the ego, we live in a society surrounded by negativity. We receive messages on what we can and cannot do and what we must do to be happy. The message, briefly, advises us to remain in our comfort zones. A clear message from the ego. At times, these messages can be seen as some sort of negative plot against our excellence. I am sure that you have met persons in your life who simply claim certain career paths or activities are "just not for them." I am sure that if you had the opportunity to hear the origin of that belief, you would hear stories about childhood, school, family life, and even about one's peers that were fraught with discouragement as opposed to supporting the individual with their dreams or ideas. (You may even relate to this!) This person continues to grow up in a society where following your dreams is discouraged, and the focus becomes all about staying in your lane and remaining comfortable. Overall, there is a focus on negativity as opposed to positivity. It all feels like some sort of evil plot by society against ensuring people can grow into their excellence. This negativity versus positivity is boxed and can be interpreted along two separate mindsets – a fixed or negative mindset versus a growth or positive mindset.

Interpretation of thoughts or sayings is governed by the mindset and surrounded by the spirit. As seen above in the parable, two servants interpreted their gift as an opportunity for growth, but one saw it as an opportunity to protect.

Seeing the ego is such a dominant force in carving our personality, is there any guidance to help us overcome the control of the ego?

Overcoming the Ego

You are the only one capable of overcoming the limitations of your ego. To do so, self-insight is essential. You may need to recalibrate your thought process, which may result in you becoming less offended by criticism. The more attention placed on criticism, the more defensive you become, which can lead to you becoming quarrelsome, with the resultant toll that has on your energy and focus.

There is no need to go through life with the persistent need to win or to be right. This may muddy the contact with your true self. Since self-reflection in this circumstance may be a blur.

Deepak Chopra advises that we must go beyond the constant clamor of ego, beyond the tools of logic and reason, to the still, calm place within us: The realm of the soul.

Though the ego is protective, it also enjoys judging and comparing others to you. We should strive to vacate the seat of superiority or inferiority. This serves no useful purpose apart from resenting others. It encourages confrontation and hostility among people. This rubs you from life's true enjoyment.

Overcoming the ego leads to a type of internal peace that is based on satisfaction. The craving for accomplishments is silenced by overcoming the ego.

Since the protection extended to us by the ego tries to keep us in our comfort zone and tries to ensure that we are safe, would there be any need to override it? Sticking to the persistence of the ego, we will not venture outside our comfort zones and will seek to keep our being from risk-taking and challenges, but unless we challenge ourselves, we do not grow. The fixed mindset is simply an enemy of personal growth.

People act in accordance with their beliefs (be it negative or positive). This is the basis by which your **mindset** is generated. Boiled down to its simplest platform, your mindset governs the way in which you manage a situation. There are two mindsets we can choose to possess: a **fixed mindset** or negative mindset and a **growth mindset or positive**. As with our bodies – our minds – also require nourishment and an optimal environment in which to flourish. There will be factors that impact our minds. We will discuss these in turn, as well as distinguish between both the fixed and growth mindsets so that you may understand which you possess and what is optimal for living a life filled with more vitality and thus help you to grow into your excellence.

Reflection:

What are some negative messages you receive daily?

Can you identify any aspect in your life which is affected by naysayers?

Now that you understand how the people around you influence you, how do you plan to address this situation?

Which do you consider is most useful in your life comfort or creativity?

_____

_____

_____

_____

_____

_____

_____

_____

_____

Let us begin with the importance of nourishing our minds for the better. We will further examine the growth and fixed mindset and come to fully understand how the mindset affects your life. I will offer you a clear reflection and guidance on taking care of your mind.

Chapter 6: Boxed In

Life is not simple; people can be boxed in as heroes or villains: Jessica Hagedorn

Society aims to fit us into a particular box. What do I mean? I hear you ask.

Whether we recognize it or not from birth, society has placed us into a group with expectations on how we are supposed to behave. We have seen the continued rebellion by babies and toddlers to confinement. Yet society continues along on its conscious or unconscious desire to box us in. This, it usually does by attaching labels to us, for example, we are told that we are smart, or we are foolish, there is no hope for us etc. These statements help to shape our mindsets by inducing a belief system in us that helps to shape our attitude to several different life experiences. Our attitude emanates from a belief system which cultivates a type of behavior that evolves into a habit from which a personality type develops. In this scenario results are amplified or explained. One may argue that through the application of labels, society has expectations of us. Unfortunately for those applying labels, a person's true potential is unknown and cannot be known, because it is unlikely for someone else to be able to predict what you can become with years of passion, hard work, support, and guidance.

Yet we see this practice flourish in society. We have an unconscious but active desire to place persons into groups. Parents, for example, will place their children in a group either inadvertently or willingly. From the simple refence of our children as being smart, the comparison begins, I am smart, because of what my parents told me. Does that therefore mean that I am smarter and thus superior to little Johnnie? If we hold on to this thought, with time, it becomes our belief and so we develop the habit (belief held for a relatively long time) which will merge into a personality type and a mindset. So, by the simple, maybe idle chatter to the little ones about how smart they are can have some pervasive consequences in how he/she feels about themself and how he/she responds to challenges. It may also define the amount of effort expended to complete a task. It may be seen that because he is smart, he does not have to try and when or if he does poorly, he either tries to explain his short comings by blaming something or someone but never himself, alternatively he may tell himself that because 'he has it', he does not have to try. For clarity let us view the impact of this language on two individuals and the impact it may have on them. (a) Say Melissa is showered with sweet nothingness about how smart she is, that may eventually lull her into believing that she must accept the label and behave in the manner expected from the label that has been applied to her. She must act in a manner to give credence to the label. She is boxed in! Mindset creation, the development of a fixed mindset. As a result, any time she is faced with a challenge or potential failure, since that goes against her belief system, (She is smart, she does not have to try) she tries to avoid the challenge, she needs to reassure herself that she is smart. Failure is not an option. Melissa needs to preserve the hand that she believes that she has been dealt, that hand 'smartness', must be validated by her actions and behavior. So, your entire being is about self-revalidation, consciously or unconsciously you go forth embarking on this journey in which you subscribe to the label placed on you, you try to protect that label. On the other hand, unlike Melissa, if Johnnie has done something well instead of telling him how smart he is and that he is obviously talented. Show recognition for his effort. Something like well-done Johnnie, I like your effort in completing the task, I am impressed. The difference being, Melissa will leave with the view that she is smart, (her talent being 'smartness') whereas the message to Johnnie, briefly, is clear, you are able to achieve with effort. This will help Johnnie accept that to achieve there must be effort. So, though he has the raw material needed to succeed, he needs to try. I refer you back to the parable above in Chapter 5 of the talents/gifts received by the servants. In the case of the servant who received the one talent, his immediate desire was to protect it and in so doing he buried it. By labelling individuals what are we burying?

The Phenomenon of Tiptoeing

If we accept that by labelling individuals, we are burying somethings, we will understand that to move out from this burial box, we need to break through, this thought has been expressed in numerous ways by many, we hear talk about breaking through the proverbial glass ceiling etc. which may be another way of referring to breaking through the box, a phenomenon much like tiptoeing. You see with tiptoeing you need a base, the balls of your feet but with your heels raised; the effect is a small gain in height, sufficient to crash that proverbial glass ceiling. Looked at another way, having that base you have a starting point from which you, through tiptoeing can grow. So by approaching the little ones with effort centric praise as opposed to an innate factor that you may suggest they possess, such as talent which is equivalent to labels, we may see a drift away from being boxed in and we may come to understand that the gifts or talents that we have been dealt is a mere template from which to grow, hence the creation of a different mindset, not that you are endowed with unchangeable characteristics but rather you have the necessary raw materials which through the exercise of passion, hard work, support, and guidance you can morph into anything your heart desires, thus demonstrating the growth mindset and allowing you to grow into your excellence. No one has accurate self-insight into their assets and limitations. Though I posit that one can grow using the raw materials with which he/she is endowed, it is obvious that in the process of growth you need guidance, support, training, belief, and commitment that it can be done. With this belief system you will be able to convert life setbacks into future successes.

It makes sense that with the culture of applying labels, not only are we boxing in individuals we are also burying opportunities. I believe that my former student Doctor Pastor Miles Munroe was right when he spoke of the cemetery as being the wealthiest place on earth. Why do I hear you ask? It is simply because buried within the box, the walls of the cemetery are dreams unfulfilled, opportunities not explored, books not written, and talents not developed.

The mind is a potent component of your being and a necessary component of the Triune. Even though it is carried around on the body, it directs the body's activities, so it is important that we are honest with it and nourish it appropriately, if we are to grow into our excellence.

The Power of Praise

Praising an individual is inevitable, not only can it encourage, but it also ensures recognition for the task. We must ask ourselves what we are giving praise too, the effort or the result? We all need encouragement and acknowledgement for what we do. Looking at it in this manner may have a penetrating discomfort based on the way the praise is issued and what is praised. If your praise is result based, the evidence is that this type of praise boxes you in, analogous to attachment of labels, the result is a fixed mindset, In Johnnie's case, the praise is effort based and he comes to appreciate the value of effort and so admires a challenge, the creation of a different mindset, the growth mindset, a necessary disposition to facilitate you growing into your excellence.

We are therefore saying that praise does not box you in, what boxes you is what is being praised; are you praising result and silently tying it to talent or are you praising the approach and appreciating the effort involved to get there?

The danger of praising results and making it seem that you are a natural, that you seem to have a certain gift or talent has the ill effect of stereotyping you and therefore boxes you in with a certain type of mindset that expects a certain type of behavior from you. This is not only limiting but it causes you not to expend effort to allow you to grow into your excellence. Your effort is spent trying to live according to your understanding of what that label or stereotype expects from you. You are trying to live the life someone has carved out for you. In trying to live someone's expectation of you, you fail to live your reality and in so doing your behavior mirrors what is expected from that stereotype/label. Your actions, including lying, is designed to maintain that stereotype. If the stereotype is positive your activity is designed to try to maintain it, if it is a negative label, you become fearful of deserving it.

This labelling therefore keeps you in a state of anxiety, fearful that the results of your activity may either cause you to lose your place in that stereotyped position, if the stereotype can be seen as positive or if the results of your activity don't quite lead to results that is expected in that stereotypes space, it may lead to a sense of worthlessness and a lack of belongingness.

Stereotyping is the offspring of prejudice. This thought is only based on someone's view of you and must not be supported by the choices you make. The approach to this prejudice by the growth mindset is different. It is met with confidence, and you see it as a challenge which your abilities will allow you to surmount.

The Tentacles of Our Creation

As is evident from the discussion above, we are a product of the interplay between our genetics, colloquially referred to as our DNA and our environment. An interaction between Nature and Nurture. Obviously as we grow older, our environment should have a greater role in who we become, but we know or expect a seed to give rise to the plant from which it arose. So, though the plant is the product of the seed, the seed is the important predecessor of the plant, but not only that the seed is dependent on its immediate environment to blossom and grow into a plant. Similarly, our mindset develops because of the interplay between our pluripotential raw material with which we are born and how it is nourished.

As family, teachers, coaches, and support personnel, we may be guilty of massaging the little ones with pleasantries which unknowingly leads to the creation of the mindset which when fully developed extends its tentacles to all aspects of their lives. This phenomenon, an integral and necessary component of the triune, directs and guides who we become. Through the extension of its tentacles, it influences every aspect of our person rightly or wrongly. It determines how we interpret what we see, it determines how we interact with people in the workspace, it determines how we respond to life challenges and irrespective how we present ourselves to the world, it directs the outcome. This is therefore very pervasive, and we need to be able to understand its' role to allow us to grow into our greatness.

Reflection:

_____

_____

_____

_____

Chapter 7: Nourishment of the Mind

"True silence is the rest of the mind, and is to the spirit what sleep is to the body, nourishment and refreshment" – William Penn

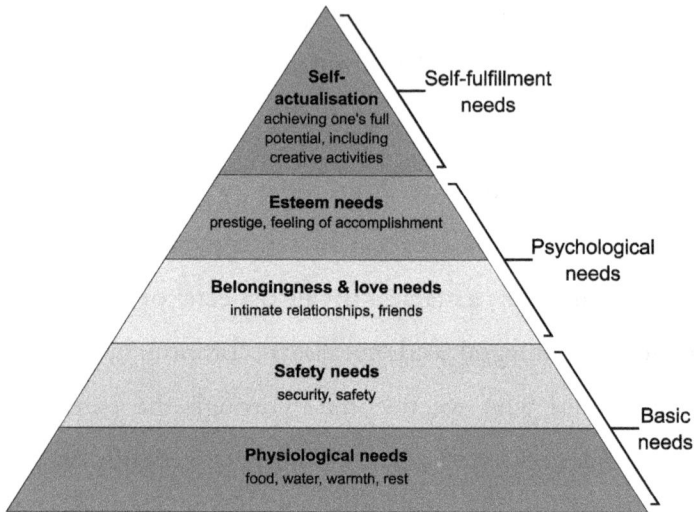

Let us revisit Maslow's hierarchy of needs. As we understand each level of the pyramid must be addressed before you can continue to move up to a higher round, and finally to the top, which is "Self-Actualization. You have addressed your physiological needs, so now we must go on to your mind.

Repeatedly in this modern era, we can no longer regard good health as just 'the absence of illnesses. With the emergence of positive psychology, evidence is unfolding that positive thinking is good for physical health, mental health, relationships, and performance in all aspects of life. Unfortunately, there is no one plaster solution to negative mindset, nor is there a magic wand to wave to convert a negative mindset to a positive mindset. The change from having a negative mindset to a positive mindset is a process which requires time and effort. The change is worth the effort for a negative mindset individual sees difficulty with every opportunity while a positive mindset individual sees the opportunity in every difficulty.

When I talk about nourishing the mind I am not talking about eating vegan and ensuring you are drinking enough water. It has nothing to do with what you put in your stomach. Because we are referring to the mind, I will be discussing your belief systems and your thoughts. Afterall, your thoughts are the foundation of your belief system. You must remember that "truths" to you are nothing but beliefs which you hold on to, and these beliefs contribute to your mindset.

Fixed Mindset and Growth Mindset

Your thought processes create a basis for nourishment of the mind. Your mind will react appropriately to how we speak to it, and how we speak to it is influenced by our mindset. There are two distinguishable mindsets that are prevalent in people: fixed mindset and growth mindset. With a **fixed mindset (as in the story of the talents above, the servant who buried his talent)**, the individual believes that their basic abilities, intelligence, and talents are fixed traits. With a **growth mindset (again as in the story of the talents above, the servants who doubled their talents)**, individuals believe that their abilities and intelligence is developed with effort, learning and ambition. Nourishing your mindset comes down to your mental

75

attitude, be it simply a positive attitude or negative one. It is of utmost importance that you understand the voice of the positive mindset so that you may be able to adapt its suggestions to nourish your mind well.

An individual with a fixed mindset is stuck and has no desire for growth or improvement. They believe, as in the story of the talents in Chapter 5, that they can only lose, so they avoid challenging themselves and aim to remain in their comfort zone.

They blame their shortcomings on their perceived lack of talent and ability. The operative reaction is to always place blame on someone or something else and to never accept responsibility for their life or truly learn (therefore grow) from the process. It is not surprising that individuals with a fixed mindset tend to be associated with a negative mental attitude. Reflecting on the Parable of Talents, we can see clearly that the third servant who received one talent had a fixed mindset. When his master questioned him, the servant offered excuses for his failure and was judged as wicked and lazy. Now, I am not saying that those who have fixed mindsets are wicked and lazy! But by not attempting to grow or explore their potential, they are robbing society of the benefit of being exposed to their talents and achievements.

As Albert Einstein said, "Nothing happens until something moves," so would it not be safe to call someone lazy because they remain in their comfort zone and are not willing to move out of their comfort zone? It is useful to observe that when one has a fixed mindset one usually doesn't take responsibility for their shortcomings. Again, you remain locked in a cycle governed by a belief system that not only does not serve you, but it can also keep you from happiness and living a fuller life. This way of operating is quite different from having a growth mindset.

When one possesses a growth mindset you believe in your abilities and intelligence and are willing to challenge yourself by developing them further. You have greater drive and will persevere in the face of setbacks. You accept mistakes as small challenges that offer you an opportunity to improve. A growth mindset is nourished through effort-oriented praise from a leader in your life.

When you possess a growth mindset, you look for opportunities to develop yourself. You readily jump into further education or training based on your needs knowing that you will be better at it overall. When you possess a growth mindset you will exude positivity. Your positive energy not only lights you up, but also lights up people around you. You see a situation with a "glass half full" attitude and therefore dedicate yourself to continue growing and taking full responsibility for yourself to make the glass full.

How to Repair a Fixed Mindset and Nourish a Growth Mindset

Dr Sonja Lyubomirsky's research indicates that 40% of our ability to sustain happiness and positivity is made possible by three skills: (a) Our ability to reframe an experience into a more positive interpretation, (b) our ability to experience gratitude and (c) our choice to be kind and generous. Research clearly shows that the mere shifting of your focus from the negative aspects in your life to more positive ones will promote happiness and well-being.

The more one tries to avoid negative thoughts and feelings the more it impinges on our mental space even against our wishes. Unfortunately, throughout our growth we focus more on the negative than the positive. This is a survival trait that we have learnt. Luckily, we can learn to shift our focus from negative to positive.

You may now be asking yourself how you can repair or help a fixed mindset, especially if you tend to operate from that place. First recognize and take comfort that a fixed mindset is not in constant operation and has triggers. These triggers can look like challenges, setbacks, challenging work, criticism, and the success of others. These triggers limit your potential when you are in a fixed mindset as you meet them with defeat and excuses as opposed to the willingness to try harder (that we see in a growth mindset). As with so many things in life, you can help yourself and change a fixed mindset.

Here are manageable steps to fighting back against the fixed mindset within yourself:

1. Be willing to learn your fixed mind set voice and engage it in conversation. I am sure you have had an experience where you think of trying something new but immediately, you start having thoughts of why it should or should not be done. The fixed mindset will encourage you to remain in your comfort zone, while your growth mindset will encourage you to see ways in which you can perform the task. Even if you do not

have the skill set, your growth mindset will encourage you to find the help you require to move forward.

2. Always be aware that you have a choice. If you can identify the voice of your fixed mindset, you can silence it and remember that you have the choice to move forward. You can avoid the negative thoughts associated with a fixed mindset by creating a mental distraction, and hence silence the voice of the negative mind set. This may require physical distraction.

3. Recognize the point of view of the growth mindset voice and as you engage the fixed mindset in conversation, you must be prepared to employ the growth mindset voice. Finding a positive friend can also be helpful when the negative thoughts of a fixed mindset visits or alternatively you could reflect on associated positives. If you are dominated with the negative thoughts of a fixed mindset, you could snap out of those thoughts by creating a list and then throwing it away. It provides useful distraction and may allow you to reflect on the negative thoughts more deeply. You must be prepared to ask yourself the question "why?" and be willing to reflect on what will happen to you if you listen to your fixed mindset voice or are willing to go forward with your growth mindset.

4. Once you recognize the growth mindset voice, be prepared to take the growth mindset advice. And its advice is usually simple: "You should do it because it is possible."

5. You must show gratitude and appreciation for what you have. Put less focus on what you do not have. It does not matter what you are grateful for, how big or small. You may wish to show gratitude by recognizing the role others play in your good fortune and well-being. It allows you to take pleasure in life's small joys. This can help you to focus on the now; and magnetizes your desire allowing you to attract appropriate vibrations and move you up the emotional positioning system (EPS) towards **level 1.**

N.B. A single expression of gratitude to another person can boost your mood for a month or more. For gratitude to have a long-lasting effect on your daily happiness, It is advisable to incorporate gratitude into your everyday life. Creating a gratitude Journal or letter will facilitate this process.

The Dangers of Fixed Mindset

People with a fixed mindset have very particular traits and shortcomings. They see challenges in their life as a barrier rather than an opportunity. Because of this they rarely excel at anything as they would rather invest their energies into looking smart rather than investing in being smart. When the fixed mindset is in the driver's seat you are filled with excuses and blame as opposed to taking responsibility for your own shortcomings. As you can imagine or may have personally experienced, this mindset keeps one stagnant. It virtually keeps you on a treadmill: your surroundings change but you remain unchanged. It is no wonder why people who constantly allow their minds to have these limits are never pioneers and rarely leaders in this world.

One of my favorite stories that demonstrates the power of overcoming a fixed mindset is that of Sir Roger Gilbert Bannister and his contribution to the sport of long-distance running. Prior to 1954, no human being living, or dead had run a mile in under four minutes, it was the popular view that it was too great a feat for a human being. It was thought of as impossible, and the view was that it could not be done. Then, despite this common belief, Roger Bannister ran a sub-four-minute mile in the 1954 Helsinki Olympics. Just knowing this feat was possible dramatically changed many athletes from having a fixed mindset to a growth mindset. Today, over 400 American athletes (including high school students!) have run sub-4-minute mile. Steve Scott, an American middle-distance runner has individually run a sub-4 minute mile 137 times. This exemplifies the power of proper "nourishment" The **IT IS POSSIBLE NOURISHMENT** with which you feed your mind.

In the example of running the sub-4-minute mile the only thing that changed was the belief system. The mile is still the same distance. Athletes are still human beings! Except in 1954, it was demonstrated that it is possible. The belief system and thus the mindset brought forth this change. With this clear example I am sure you now have many personal moments when your beliefs have tricked you into staying in a fixed mindset. The only way to really revive your mind and ensure you stay on track to living a long and vibrant life is to nourish your growth mindset. Without it you will remain stuck and never realize your full potential.

Reflection:

Based on the evidence above, do I operate from a growth or fixed mindset?

What three things I can do right now in my life to nourish a growth mindset?

Can I think of someone in my life who has a growth mindset?

What are their defining traits?

_____

_____

_____

_____

_____

_____

_____

What other supports can you employ to continue to nourish your mind? Look at your environment and the respective messages. You can choose to appropriately nourish your mind to facilitate a growth mindset or to hold onto the fixed mindset and continue to blame others for your shortcomings. Now that you are aware of this, your decision now becomes informed.

Chapter 8: How Your Environment Affects Your Mind

"What lies behind you and what lies in front of you, pales in comparison to what lies inside of you." - Ralph Waldo Emerson

When you wake up in the morning you may have a truly clear intention of how you want to approach your day. You may feel confident and ready to take on all the tasks and work at hand. As the day progresses it becomes clear that stimuli designed with ulterior purposes are constantly coming at you, and not all of them are constructive. We live in a world in which our influences are negative and so we must actively work to make a change. For example, people may offer well-intentioned advice because they feel it is in your best interest. However, it is coming from their own belief systems. You may come across people who are constantly blaming others or circumstances for their own stagnation.

Be it our own family, co-workers, or strangers with whom we cross paths, the people that surround us can create a corrosive and negative environment in which it is a struggle to nurture our mind in positive ways. Let us examine ways in which you can keep your surroundings more positive which will feed into your inspiration and nurture a growth mindset.

Neutralizing An Environment Hostile To Your Mind

Understanding how to neutralize the negativity that surrounds you is an essential skill if you wish to continue reviving your mind and stay on the path to realizing your full potential and living a life full of vitality. Again, I cannot stress enough that if your body is catered to, but your mind suffers, you cannot have access to adding years to our life and life to our years. All parts of your person are connected.

Some may suggest that you just simply ignore the negativity and go on with your day. However, that is easier said than done! No matter your efforts, the adverse chatter will always get through to you.

First, I recommend that you clarify your priorities in life. Is it to follow through on some important goals or remain very present so that you can create some new goals. When you have a clear idea of what your priorities are you can then work on removing clutter from your life that interferes with your ability to reach these goals. This will include identifying people in your life with fixed mindsets and work on creating distance or removing them all together from your environment, this may include reducing the time spent around them or eliminating them from your core group of associates. You must be prepared to walk away.

These people may be family and friends. You must be willing to manage a bit of emotional fallout if you remove yourself from particular social circles that no longer serve the growth of a more positive mind. Criticism may be directed at you for a change in your behavior, but again you must work on ensuring that the naysayers do not infiltrate your thought processes and belief systems. Stay grounded and strong knowing that you are creating the best life you can for yourself.

I am not recommending that you become asocial. Human beings are sociable, I am just suggesting that you become more selective in choosing your friends and associates. You may choose to have distinct categories of associates. For example, there may be people who you may choose to share a joke or play games with, but from whom you will not seek guidance or advice. You have come to realize that they have negative mindsets, and their contribution will not nourish your mindset and provide it with the appropriate environment in which to blossom. It is about understanding your relationships and the ones that appropriately feed you.

Nourishing "Food" For The Mind

Your mind is nourished by the thoughts that are a product of your mindset. Cultivating your growth mindset is a dynamic daily undertaking and the process is determined by the nourishment you provide. This nourishment is your thoughts, which create the environment in which you allow your mindset to develop.

When beginning your day there are simple steps to start it on the right footing:

- **Positive affirmations:** This is positive self-talk in which you continuously encourage yourself to see the glass as half full rather than half empty.

- **Instill in your belief system that everything is possible:** This will cultivate a new thought pattern so when facing a challenge, you no longer will say to yourself that it is impossible. Instead, you will remember that it *is* possible and immediately start thinking of ways in which you may overcome the challenge. Whether you choose to go through the challenge or around the challenge, believe you me there is always a way to overcome it!

- **Understand and recognize that no one person knows it all:** This includes you. Yes, sometimes it requires tapping into the expertise of others. Be prepared to learn! Appreciate the value of mentorship and remember that everything is possible!

- **Challenges or negativity will cross your path:** Be prepared to recognize them, confront them, and manage them while keeping a cheerful outlook throughout your day. Even when you do not feel ready for them, you can get through it!

As you go about your business, always make a commitment to remain neutral in situations or to leave an environment more positive than before you entered it. Create a strong focus on positive experiences no matter how small they are. This commitment to constantly connect to the brightness of your day feeds the growth mindset.

Having a sense of humor is necessary! Not only will it further safeguard you from the negativity you will encounter, but it will also strengthen your will. Your challenges will show up throughout the day. You will need to escape from negative moments. You will be confronted with your own failures and shortcomings, but you will be more willing to learn from them. Never forget each failure is an opportunity for learning and support for your growth mindset and is a step closer to your desired goal.

Continue to focus on the present. The past is gone and cannot be retrieved. We can never change what has happened in our lives. All we can control is how we react to the present and the choices we make. This is most important in nurturing your mind in a positive way. Connect with the now, as it is all you have.

My Story

Throughout this chapter, we have lamented the volume of negativity which surrounds us daily. Our parents, our siblings, our schoolteachers, and those who we come across in our day-to-day activities. Their negativity is conspiring against us, as if there is a sinister plot discouraging us from dreaming or moving from our comfort zones. In fact, many believe that the cemetery is the wealthiest place on the planet, since within it lies the frustrated dreams, the unwritten New York Times best sellers, the undeveloped potential invention which the conspirators have been able to silence and rob the world from ever experiencing.

Repeatedly, we must find some way of shutting out the chatter. Had the Wright brothers been swayed by the negativism of the day, they would have never developed and flew the first airplane, an invention which you will agree has succeed figuratively in making the world smaller; Had Alexander Graham Bell listened to the distracting noises, he would have never succeeded in pioneering the development of our telephone system, an invention, you will agree, which has succeeded in bringing us together even if we are apart. Had Eric Yuan listened to the naysayers, his development of Zoom video conferencing software, would have never occurred and the world would have been robbed of this much needed communication tool which proved priceless during the Coronavirus pandemic. Thus, giving new meaning to the apparent hitherto meaningless phrase "apart but still together." The world continues to benefit from the efforts of those who filter out the naysayers and allow them to have a limited impact on their activities.

I have been exposed to my fair share of naysayers and I have tried a myriad of ways to avoid the noise. Try as we may there is noise that tends to get through. This noise may be very damaging with a long-lasting impact. I want to share two such examples from my own life with you of brief statements made to me during my teenage years which have had a profound impact on me and the way in which my life has unfolded.

At high school in year 10 I worked hard at my academics as I always did. My overall year position was second among all year 10 students at my school. My form Mistress at the time, in her end of year comments wrote: 'Harris has the ability but prides himself as the clown of the class.' The teacher was our history teacher, a trusted and respected influence. I had scored an A+ in history during that semester, but that did not matter much; I had forgotten much of what I learnt in her classes, but these comments lived with me; the damage had been done. I loved comedy and loved to ensure that the people with whom I interacted were happy or at least laughing. In fact, looking back, I could have explored comedy as a career. From that comment, I thought comedy was a terrible thing, the language used, 'clown' shattered any prospect of me pursuing comedy as a career, the damage was done. It discouraged the development of my comedic skills. The result, the world of comedy and the planet has lost a willing comedian.

Equally important is the noise or chatter that knowingly or unknowingly has a positive impact. During my teenage years, I must admit that I was not focused on any specific career path. Academically, I performed creditably but I also had a keen interest in sports, specifically cricket. In fact, I made the national under 19 trials in cricket in two successive years, one year as an opening batsman and wicket keeper and the second year as a spin bowler and number 3 batsman. I was okay. I also dabbled in chicken farming and through my methods, my chief and better-established competitor sold all his birds to me and closed his chicken farm.

In the dynamic phase of my teenage years, whilst returning home from a cricket game in which I scored many runs and batted throughout the day without the loss of my wicket. My eldest brother who was a spectator at the games got home before me and told our parents about my performance. On reaching home, my father took a long hard, almost piecing look at me and said, 'Son, it seems that whatever you put your mind too, you are better than average.' I don't know the intention of that statement, but it was definitely not a frivolous comment. I have held onto that statement dearly through the years. I gain both solace and fight from it. Based on the belief that my father knew me better than any other person living or dead, made that observation, I have believed it, and it has helped me.

Granted my father departed this life about three decades ago but his words have been sacred to me and continues to live within me. Whenever I face a challenge, that may seem insurmountable, I reflect on those words to spur me forward. I remind myself that since my father knew me better than most will ever know me, and he thinks that I am better than average, then I am not average. This had the invisible power of granting me the 'can do' aura which has helped me to both consciously and unconsciously put a bit more effort in, knowing that I am better than average. With this mantra I have overcome countless challenges, irrespective of the effort required.

So, you see a kind word can move you forward, allowing you to climb high hills trying to get home. A harsh word, on the other hand, is like a dagger, killing dreams and flushing them to the cemetery which Myles Munroe considers to be the wealthiest place on the planet.

Surround yourself with others who are dedicated to living their life with a growth mindset. Cultivate friendships with more positive people who understand the importance of nourishing the mind in a positive manner and are on board putting these practices into place themselves but are also there to support you. If possible, you may want to change work environments as well. Working on a team or in an office where people are in line with your values can be a game changer. Ideally surrounding yourself with people who have achieved what you seek is among the strongest contributors to the attainment of your goal.

Reflection:

When have I come into a negative environment and had to work on staying positive?

How did it make me feel?

Are there any specific environments in my life that I feel promote a fixed mindset as opposed to nourishing a growth mindset? Can I act?

What is something I can commit to doing every day to help myself nourish a growth mindset?

_____

_____

_____

_____

_____

_____

_____

_____

We have examined factors which nourish your mind. As you can see, sometimes it can be grand but at other times it can be a subtle word from someone you respect and believe. It depends on your mindset and where you are in the day so that you can make the best decisions. Also, keep in mind that each day is different, and your process may have to change daily depending on what is happening in your life. But I know with practice and dedication you will be able to surmount the challenges you will face. Again, it is all about taking responsibility and to be willing to stay on the course.

To ensure you have a complete set of tools that will allow your growth mindset to flourish, let us dig into aspects of our lives which negatively impact our minds. It is always important to study the insightful and the dull so that you can empower yourself to make the best and most informed choices in reviving your mind.

Chapter 9: Factors That Impact Your Mind

"I have learned over the years that when one's mind is made up, this diminishes fear; knowing what must be done does away with fear" -Rosa Parks

There are varying views out there on how your mind functions in your life. It may be a task-based mechanism that runs on its own, while it may be viewed as relatively labile, constantly bouncing back and forth between negative (fixed) and positive (growth) states depending on what is at hand. As I have expressed, I like to think that we have the potential for both fixed and growth mindsets, and that these mindsets are influenced by both innate sources and our external environment. We were all born with the tools necessary to excel in at least one thing. However, the possibility of excelling at a plethora of things may be available to you depending on your mindset and how you face the challenges around and within you. How your life unfolds is directly dependent on the factors you welcome into your life which influences your mindset.

Let us first examine the external factors that you are constantly up against when attempting to keep your mindset positive and in a growth state. Firstly, we have the **negative environment** which we discussed fully in the previous chapter. So, let's jump to the second and third factors: **bad habits** and **limiting beliefs**.

Bad Habits

To put it simply, bad habits are activities that you constantly engage in that add little or no true value to your life. When you engage in your unhealthy habits you squander your time, begin procrastinating and miss deadlines and goals. I am sure you already understand or have a good sense of unhealthy habits that steal your time. If you do not, I recommend you begin journaling, that is recording how you spend *all* your time. Audit your daily schedule for every activity you engage in including playing video games, watching TV, going out for drinks with friends etc. Analyze how your time has been spent after a week and see if there are any unhealthy habits that you have unknowingly developed that are robbing you of productive, goal orientated activities.

I am not suggesting that you never take breaks. Of course! We have talked about exercising temperance and the value of rest. I want you to be empowered and learn how to eliminate your bad habits. *How* you spend your time will make a world of difference and set you up for a more inspiring mindset. Getting closer to achieving your dreams starts with awareness and choosing to engage in more productive activities that contribute directly to your goals.

Limiting Beliefs

We grow up in a world in which our parents, teachers, and society believe in what they tell us. However, the things they must teach us are invariably negative limiting beliefs masquerading as guidance. Now, to be fair to our parents and others who we look up to (mine included), they only shared what they knew, and they believed this guidance to be true. By this our predecessor's own limiting beliefs move to a new generation and further spreads. If beliefs are long standing thoughts, and your beliefs feed into your mindset which subsequently feed the mind, you can appreciate the potential impact of limiting beliefs that you may have.

Advice offered to you throughout your life may sow the seeds of accepted limitations in your mindset which short-change your future and encourage the development of a fixed mindset. Future leaders may hold beliefs about themselves that simply are not true, or they are not willing to try to further themselves because of these held beliefs. For example, a future leader may have a held belief of, "I am not good at Mathematics", and would never think to pursue any sort of studies in mathematics. When you fall into this sort of habitual thought pattern of limiting yourself to what you think you are good at and bad at, it will constantly hinder your growth potential. You may come up against challenges and be willing to give up as opposed to appreciating the challenge and attempting to overcome it. That is a fixed mindset vs growth mindset at play.

A strong boundary to the external factors of a negative environment, unhealthy habits and limiting beliefs is required or they will push up against your positive or growth mindset. You must be keenly aware of them and willing to continuously adjust yourself so that you can keep them from damaging your growth mindset. Let us now examine the **internal** influences that will challenge you from the inside out. One may argue that they are products of external influences but they are marginally different. Let's examine **fear, boredom** and

stress.

Reflection:

What bad habits can I immediately identify when examining how I spend my time?

How are these bad habits keeping me from my goals?

Are there any limiting beliefs that I keep pushing up against?

Are there any limiting beliefs that I can identify that stem from my childhood?

What sources are feeding me limiting beliefs right now that I do not need to engage with?

_____

_____

_____

_____

_____

_____

_____

_____

_____

Fear

This is an acronym which perfectly defines fear.

F.E.A.R.: **F**alse **E**xpectations **A**ppearing **R**eal.

Fear is crippling and stops you from moving forward. It rarely visits your mind alone and usually comes accompanied by its friend Regret: "I could've...", "I would've..." Thus, a vicious cycle is created as fear will stop you from moving forward with dreams and goals, and when you do not follow through on what your heart and mind desires, you are left with a knot of regret in your stomach. Fear is a major cause of procrastination, which is a thief of your precious time. It leads to a fixed mindset and causes you to blame everything and everyone but yourself. When you are in a fear cycle it can reveal to you that you have lost your will, you are out of control, and prevent further engagement with your life and aspirations.

Chemically, your fear can have a sinister effect on your brain by impairing formation of long-term memories and damaging parts of the brain such as the hippocampus (a player in your learning and memory). This can lead to diminishing the function of regulating fear which can result in you being perpetually anxious. Being in a constant state of anxiety can obviously hinder your growth mindset. If you suffer from chronic fear, you will require professional help to have an opportunity to live a dynamic and fruitful life. This is how damaging fear can be.

You must appreciate fear is not necessarily bad and in fact, can be very protective. When you are in actual danger, fear will advise you how to stay safe and alive. However, you must also understand fear can be created because of internal constructs for which there is no basis. Fear is crippling and can influence your abilities and decisions. This fear may be particularly difficult to overcome, and often requires the help of professionals (such as trained therapists) to help you through your fear slowly until you overcome it.

Growing up, I had a severe case of Nyctophobia (I was afraid of the dark). I don't know what led to the germination of that fear, but it may have arisen from stories that we were told of unsavory characters lurking in the dark who are able to see you but you are unable to see them. These stories had a significant impact on me growing up and caused me to avoid dark spaces and even now as an adult, I still get a creepy feeling when I enter dark spaces. With time, I have become less scared about entering dark spaces, but the diminution of my fear did not merely come about by me getting older. I went into dark spaces repeatedly with someone holding my hand till I was able to demonstrate that I was less fearful of the dark and can now enter dark spaces with less fear than I did previously. I must confess though that occasionally, I still do experience hair raising anxiety on entering dark spaces.

Reflection:

How does fear show up in my life?

When was the last time I let fear stop me from moving forward with something?

Can I recall the last time I experienced a cycle of fear? How did it impact my life at the time?

_____

_____

_____

_____

_____

_____

_____

Boredom

Like fear, boredom is internally generated and is a negative emotion you may experience daily. Now, a particular state of boredom may be beneficial when you are trying to work creatively as it can stimulate your imagination etc. However, for the sake of focusing on how you can safeguard your mindset we will just explore the type of boredom that can adversely affect your mind (even kill you). A helpful way to examine this is to understand that there are two distinct personality types that tend to suffer from boredom.

The first are people who have an impulsive personality type.

They constantly need new experiences and find the world to be chronically under stimulating. This causes not only a sense of boredom but also anxiety and mental strain. So, imagine that you have this personality type. You constantly need new experiences or stimulation in one way or another. Just simply going about a routine does not feel good to you. You may perceive things to be boring or find yourself reacting because things just do not seem exciting enough. This boredom is not healthy because it causes you to constantly be reactive and not being able to be in the present. You constantly look to the future as opposed to being able to remain in the present.

The second personality type finds the world at large to be a very fearful place. To remain comfortable, they will tend to shut themselves in and always stay within their comfort zone. Of course, these people may feel unsatisfied with life and find their day-to-day life boring. This type of boredom may be self-inflicted. So, now imagine you are this personality type. You constantly live in fear and deny yourself from having any adventure in your life. You like to keep things under control. You aim to keep things under control so that you can remain comfortable. Of course this brings about a sense of boredom. The unknowing moments in life can be the most exciting. If you are not out there living in an unknown future, then you will feel unsatisfied with your carefully curated reality.

Regardless of the personality type, these constant feelings of boredom can cause people to harm themselves. This may take the form of smoking, drinking excessive alcohol, comfort eating and experimenting with illegal drugs. It is all an effort to alleviate boredom and try to make things more exciting or try to self soothe. On a grander scale, boredom is strongly associated with depression and destructive behavior. The popular Whitehall Study done in the UK confirmed that people who were most likely to get bored were 30% more likely to die within 3 years! (This is not in line with the revival of oneself and adding years to your life and life to your years!). For one to break the boredom cycle and thrive, you need to identify the behavior, eradicate it and work on replacing it with a behavior that is more positive and productive. This is a big job especially if you have been feeling this boredom for years, but it is vital to break your relationship with boredom so that you can develop a positive mindset.

The cycle of boredom can be broken by just shaking up your routine and changing the way in which you do things. The cycle can be broken by changing your environment. Knowing the reasons for boredom may go a long way in breaking the cycle. The boredom would be the result of engaging in the habit of procrastination or you may be stuck in doing monotonous tasks. Could it be that your boredom is the result of lack of energy, direction, or focus? There is insufficient mental stimulation, you do not feel sufficiently challenged. Whatever the cause of your boredom, it is within them you will find the clue to break the cycle.

Reflection:

Do I ever find myself bored?

What is my personality type?

Do I identify at all with being impulsive and needing stimulus all the time?

Do I need to try to be in control and stay safe?

How can I combat boredom in my own life?

_____

_____

_____

_____

_____

_____

_____

_____

Stress

The last internal influence on your mindset that I will discuss is stress. Stress is an enigma when it comes to its influence on your mindset. Stress is seen from both a fixed and growth mindset. When you are in a growth mindset stress is a welcome challenge and an opportunity to gain experience. On the contrary when you are in a fixed mindset, stress can lead to negative cognitive and physiological outcomes. Stress in your life may cause sleep disturbances and psychological and emotional strain leading to confusion, anxiety, and depression. In extreme cases, stress can even manifest as a psychotic illness.

The value of stress is dependent on the impact it has on your person. Stress modulates mindset. If you possess a growth mindset, you will see stressful situations as an opportunity to try harder. You will feel encouraged to make things happen or even to get help, thereby managing stress efficiently and effectively. Whereas if you have a fixed mindset, you are more likely to fail at managing stress. You may see stress as a sort of punishment or even as an indicator that you do not belong or cannot achieve your goal. In more extreme cases, individuals may see stress as a reason to succumb. I am sure you are familiar with or have heard of stories in which an individual simply gives up on life by committing suicide and uses the stresses they are experiencing as a motivator to end their life. Therefore, to ensure that your mind stays on a path of revival and vitality, it is essential to manage stress in your life effectively.

Before we move on, I also want to briefly mention one of the most severe forms of stress and a newly described entity called Post Traumatic Stress Disorder (PTSD). Previously it was described as an individual's construct. However, professionals have now come to understand it is an extreme reaction to a large-scale stress an individual may have experienced. There are facets of PTSD which can include uncontrollable negative experiences or reactions which can impact social relationships and one's overall quality of life. If you feel that you may be suffering from any form of PTSD, I urge you to seek professional help. There are now a variety of treatments offered that can help you get your life back.

Reflection:

Do I have a healthy relationship with stress?

Are stresses in my life affecting my health in ways such as disrupting healthy sleep cycles or causing me unwanted anxiety or depression?

When I feel stress, do I feel as if it sucks the energy out of me? Or do I feel motivated for action by the stress I feel in my life?

_____

_____

_____

_____

_____

_____

_____

I hope you feel filled with inspiration as we complete this section of your full body revival. The mind is such an intricate and sensitive part of your being, but never forget that you have the power to stay positive and operate from a growth mindset. You will find that when you are able to do the work of reviving your mind, your life will seem brighter and more fulfilling. You will feel more energized and gain stamina to continue doing the work needed to add years to your life and life to years. When you work on your mind and its relationship to the world around you, your relationship to your precious life will also strengthen.

We have covered reviving your body and mind. It is now time to dive into the beauty of your spirit and how it relates to your life and the world around you. You have exciting and important work ahead!

PART 3: THE SPIRIT

'There are no constraints on the human mind, no walls around the human spirit, no barriers to our progress except those we ourselves erect." - Ronald Reagan

Humankind is a complex entity composed of a physical body, a mind, and a spirit. The interrelationship suggests that the mind is central and can impact the physical body, but the spirit oversees the mind. They all act collectively as a whole with dysfunction in any arm leading to ill health in the triune. As you may recall we refer to this as a triune, where three different entities co-exist to comprise a whole. We have examined your body which we can explore through our five senses. We have also examined your mind, which you cannot see or touch, but you can observe at work. It is now time to examine and discuss your spirit. It is the third component which makes up your person. However, it takes a bit more open-mindedness as the Spirit is observed, through our emotions as a fair indication of the status of our spirit. The presence of our spirit continues to influence your day-to-day activities.

Reflection:

How do I become aware of the working of my spirit?

Is the spirit different from the mindset?

How can I gauge the status of my spirit?

Is my emotion an indication of my spirit?

_____

_____

_____

_____

_____

_____

_____

Chapter 10: What Is the Human Spirit

"I believe very deeply in the human spirit, and I have a sense of awe about it. I look around and ask, what makes the difference? What is it? I have known people the world has thrown everything at – to discourage them, to kill them, to break their spirit! And yet something about them retains a dignity. . ." - Horton Foote

There are countless definitions of the human spirit and why it exists. Scholars have noted that there is a physical and non-physical world coexisting. The spirit is thought to be part of a vibrational energy that we cannot see, cannot create, or destroy. Some people believe that our spirit includes our intellect, emotions, fears, passions, and creativity.

There is no denying that our spirit is a part of us, it is just how to define it for yourself so that you may have a relationship with it. The spirit is like an emotion, that is, we know it exists but cannot touch it and may not be able to rationalize it. This is distinct from the mindset, although it may guide our mindset and thought process. Let me clarify. Fear is an emotion which is brought on by what our thoughts tell us, for example, if we think we are going to be attacked by a dog that will generate the emotion of fear, but is that mindset? Surely not? Is that simply a thought, of course it is but it produces an emotion.

The neuroscientist tells us that there is both a subjective and objective assessment of thought. Subjectively, the neuroscientist claims that our thoughts come from nowhere; they just pop into our heads or emerge in the form of words leaving our mouths. Objectively, our thoughts emerge from neural processes which come from everywhere. Whereas in the previous section, we learnt that our mindset is a product of our thoughts which we have held unto and as a result, this developed into a belief system which leads to our mindset that directs our activities; we recognize our thoughts have an emotional component and it is this component of our thoughts that feeds our spirit.

As we go through this section, we will learn about the existence of the emotional positioning system (EPS) which indicates the appropriateness of what is presented to our spirit. We learnt in section 2 that our thoughts nourish our mindset, the chronicity of which generates our belief system. We are now addressing the influence on our spirit by our emotions. If our thoughts are appropriate, we will tend to have our emotions moving in the direction of level 1 on the EPS.

We can therefore begin to sense the interconnectedness of the components of the triune. Our bodies, mind, and spirit acting harmoniously to produce us; the final product.

The Role of Your Spirit

You may identify your Spirit as that small voice inside you that helps you to decipher right from wrong. It is that entity one occasionally describes as your morals which guides you along the right path. Your spirit may comfort you in times of need and your very spirit may even function as an advocate. According to the bible, we are made in God's image, and God is a spirit, so it is palpably obvious then that we too have a spiritual component. But what exactly is the spirit? We cannot touch, feel, see, smell, or taste it. Is it a figment of our imagination? Surely, we can recognize the workings of the spirit which is best manifested through our emotions, and it yields or bears results or fruits. We have referred to people as having a cheerful spirit, a kind spirit, a forgiving spirit etc.; Giving credence to the view that our spirit is best reflected in our emotions.

Many believe that our spirit is linked to an authority greater than ourselves and is our way of connecting with the greater good and receiving gifts and power into our lives. The Bible says if we ask for anything, it shall be given. The teachings of Abraham-Hicks are based on the understanding that the non-physical world has an abundance to offer you, but you must ask for it. Rhonda Bryne, the author of "The Secret" approaches it from a similar but slightly different angle when she proposes we can gain whatever we ask of the universe through one of the natural laws, The Law of Attraction. Mastin Kipp (leadership coach) teaches that the number one hindrance people have working against them is that they do not believe success is possible for them. As you can see, all these ideas from great thought leaders and scripture have in common, a belief. Believing first that there is something more than just the life you can see and feel. Being willing to ask for what you want and finally believing that you shall receive it. The adage that anything the mind of man can perceive (think of) and believe, that it can achieve, looked at differently, we understand that we must first have a dream, but that is not enough, we must believe that that dream is possible (the belief is essential) but not only that it is an emotion, hence nourishment for the spirit. Because we know it is possible, our belief system takes over, our spirit is appropriately nourished, and our spirit facilitates the rendering of our request. This is identical to faith which is commonly referred to among those of a Christian persuasion.

Faith

Faith in religious circles is the substance of things hoped for, the evidence of things not seen. The literature on hope is equivocal, it says that hope is at least not a fundamental emotion because hope is situation specific and contingent on one's own abilities. Yet hoping for an item is not contingent on our own abilities and in that context therefore, hope is an emotion. By extrapolation, then, if we accept hope as an emotion, and we define faith as the substance of an emotion, faith must therefore be an emotion and hence potential nourishment for our spirit. This is almost identical to bible verse (Mark11:24) that says whatever you ask for in prayer, believe that you have received it, and it will be yours. To receive it, you must have faith, you must display the emotion of belief, the spirit must be appropriately nourished. The spirit world has boundless goodies for us to tap into, our spiritual component allows us to tap into these boundless goodies but to obtain them we must ask, believe, and exercise faith, which nourishes our spirit appropriately. Both belief and faith are emotions and are therefore potential nourishment for our spirit. If our belief and faith are aligned, then the appropriate nourishment of our spirit will result, we will then move towards position 1 on the emotional positioning system (EPS).

This is quite similar, almost identical to Abraham-Hicks's teachings but expressed very differently. Abraham-Hicks prefers to view the interaction in terms of vibrations. He implies that if our vibrations or emotions are in alignment, we will move towards the upper pole along the EPS.

Rhonda Bryne, the author of the secret, addresses the same subject and speaks of the natural Law, the Law of attraction. This law as stated claims that like attract like. Unfortunately, this law does not withstand scrutiny in the manner stated.

Since our belief system originates from our thoughts and the emotional component of our thoughts nourishes our spirit, your spirit revolves around your own belief system. You must ask yourself if you are willing to believe there is more to your life than just what you can see or feel and whether you are willing to step out of your own way, out of your comfort zone to achieve more. We are offered anything we ask of the universe. It simply says ask and you shall receive, we are chided mockingly, when we are told the reason we do not have is because we do not ask. We have no excuse but to ask, in asking however we must have faith or belief that our request shall be granted. The popular teaching that what you believe you can achieve is not far-fetched, but you must be willing to receive and to that I add, you must be prepared to give thanks. For by showing appreciation for your gifts, you encourage the universe to give more.

The Christian teachings is that when you ask, you get one of three responses: **YES, NO** or **NOT YET** (though there is no biblical support for the **NO** response). All the bible specifically states is ask, and it shall be given! Others interpret the offer differently, claiming that there is a three-step process involved. The interpretations are almost identical but the response from a request is never no. It is always given, as per the statement in the bible; ask and it shall be given.

The interpretation of the Christians **'not yet'** response is based on your level of preparedness for the receipt of the requested item. If there appears to be a delay in your receipt of the requested item, the individuals of a Christian persuasion will interpret this delay as either a **'no'** response or a **'not yet'** response. They then seek to justify their claim by indicating that the omnipotent creator did not believe you needed the item which you requested, hence the response, **'NO'**. Unfortunately, I disagree with Christian teaching here, as there is no biblical support for a **'NO'** response. The **'not yet,'** though those of a Christian persuasion may interpret this to be the result of a lack of faith! We must recall that there was no time given when your goodies which you requested from the universe would be available to you. If we ask, it will be given. Is the delay in receiving our requested goodies the result of a lack of faith?

The Christian teachings seem to suggest that the greater your faith, the more likely you will receive the request which you have made, a sort of **quid pro quo** arrangement. The biblical evidence for this is lacking.

In none of the biblical texts quoted does it say that a request

113

is put on hold. The advice has always been to ask, and it shall be given to you. To obtain clarity, I tried to question the use of shall in that statement as opposed to will. Both words talk of future events but there are two basic English rules which govern their use. Additionally, there is a division between a strong and a normal future event. Grammatically correct English uses 'shall' to address normal future events when using the first person such as I and/or We. Will is used to reflect normal future events in the second and third person (you, it, or they). In strong future events, there is an emotional attachment to the future and the roles of will and shall reversed, with this in mind let us review the statement, ask and it (third person) shall be given unto you. Inherent in that statement is the strong future that it (third person) shall be granted. Our spirit is nourished by our emotions, was it a deliberate play on words to ensure our spirit is nourished in the process? Remember the emotional component of our thoughts nourish our spirit. Note the roles are reversed so to relay the strength of the future and ensure its emotional content, the words shall is used. It is a promise laced with emotions. Interestingly, the term does not give a finite time during which your request will be granted. What we do know, however, it shall be granted. So, from the biblical promise all we can claim is that our request shall be granted but we do not know when, herein may lie the basis of the 'Not Yet' response, hence the need for both faith and patience.

Faith is the substance of things hoped for, the evidence of things not seen. A new entity, 'hope without seeing that which you requested' In other words we are asked to move beyond the physical.

114

Hope is a feeling of expectation and desire for a particular thing to happen. Taking this definition and relating it to the Christian teaching of a need for more faith would complicate interpretation by suggesting that there are degrees of feelings of expectation. Naturally, our expectations in everyday life waver, so this must be controlled to ensure we achieve what we requested if we are to avoid the **'NOT YET'** response? Other interpretations of the workings of the spirit traverse similar paths without establishing a bridge, an entity needed to elucidate the issue.

The concept of faith hints at emotion without stating so but let us look more closely at the accepted meaning of faith and analyze what it is saying. We claim that faith is the substance of things hoped for, the evidence of things not seen. We will quickly realize that hope generates an expectation, an emotion if you will, in us. Hope is fundamentally not an emotion; it is very situation specific and may be contingent on our own abilities. The second part of the definition of Faith…. the evidence of things not seen… instills within us clarity that our emotions are involved. It also injects the need for a belief. Combined we have a hope (a situation specific entity capable of generating an emotion and we have evidence, though we cannot see it, but it generates belief) and belief. So, we have a believable emotion which is tantamount to faith. Obviously, therefore, we ask (ask and it shall be given unto you) and we have the belief that we will receive, through faith (the believable emotion). Our emotions will reflect happiness which will take us towards level 1 on the EPS. This will automatically start paying us a dividend, as the happiest, most positive people tend to be the healthiest, most successful, most generous, and even the most popular. Positivity is contagious. This positivity therefore feeds back into your mindset and benefits not only you but everyone around you.

Above we mentioned that our spirit is both an advocate and a comforter, both tasks we can readily observe will make you happy. We can now appreciate the role of positive psychology, the scientific study of positive human emotion, happiness, and well-being. Emanating from this realm of science is the realization that positivity can benefit all aspects of human life and health. There is therefore an inevitable need for the contribution from the spirit if we are to benefit from the addition of years to our lives and life to our years.

Abraham-Hicks's teachings have a different take on how we receive. As per his teachings, the source of all goodies is the universe which has an inexhaustible supply. To obtain anything from this abundance, you only need to request it. Abraham-Hicks contends, though he does not reference it, that all you need to do is to make the request. He also indicates that there is a three-step process before one can accept his requested goodies:

1. The request (which is always granted, as per Abraham-Hicks)

2. The Granting of the request.

3. The receipt of the goodies.

It is at #3 that Abraham-Hicks teachings deviate from the biblical teachings. Though the bible does not give an explanation, it is obvious that if something is given, it must be received. The bible does not detail the receiving process, it leaves a void which differing interpretations fills. Abraham-Hicks seems to suggest that the void is bridged with vibrational energy, if you follow his insight on vibrational energy, according to your vibrations and the vibrations of your request.

They claim that if your vibrations and the vibrations of your request are in alignment, you will receive that for which you ask. They contend that a shift in your vibrations will give you instant emotional evidence, that is if your vibrations and the vibrations of your request are in alignment you will experience a shift in your emotional positioning system towards the pole of happiness but it won't yield instant physical evidence of the goodies you requested. Is this not the definition of faith? The evidence of things not seen!! From that standpoint Abraham-Hicks's interpretation of the process is closer to the bible's teachings than the interpretation of the Christian leadership. It also explains the delay and failure to receive the requested goodies.

Rhonda Bryne, the author of "The Secret" approaches it from a similar but slightly different angle when she proposes we can gain whatever we ask of the universe through the activity of a natural law, the law of attraction.

Mastin Kipp believes that the number-one hindrance to success is people who believe it is not possible for them. He says if you believe something is not possible, then you are right. And the whole universe will be against you, not because the universe is a bad place but because that is how you are interacting with it, and all you will look for is proof of why it is not possible.

In attempting to bridge this void all the authors quoted are saying the same thing which we will have a closer look at in this section.

The workings of the spirit within you allow great emotional characteristics to emerge which are referred to as the fruits of the spirit, all good qualities which coats you with a veneer that we should all aspire to. The fruits are love, joy, peace, forbearance, kindness, goodness, faithfulness, gentleness, and self-control. All traits, I am sure you will agree, help us to be better people and facilitate better interpersonal relationships.

If your spirit is shining forth within you, a bystander would be expected to recognize the unavoidable love that you show for your fellow man, your happiness will be clearly and readily identifiable and you would obviously be at peace with your environment, neighbors, and colleagues. The fruits of forbearance, kindness, goodness, and faithfulness are all virtues we love to see in our fellow men and with gentleness and self-control thrown in, a collection of emotions that we can display and are manifested by us in varying degrees but together makes our neighbors and associates comfortable with us. Aspiring to the acquisition of these virtues is commendable.

Reflection:

How do I identify my spirit?

When have I felt my spirit evident in my life?

When was the last time I exhibited faith in my life?

Do I show appreciation and gratitude for my gifts?

Make a list of the last five gifts for which you have been grateful.

Should I be doing things differently to really prove that I am grateful?

How may I nurture the "fruits" of spirit in my life? (love, joy, kindness, etc.)

_____

_____

_____

_____

_____

_____

_____

_____

In the following chapters of this section, I will explore how you nourish, that is cultivate and maintain these attributes, I will also explore the optimum environment in which these traits flourish and finally I will explore factors which we allow to affect our spirits.

Chapter 11: Nourishing Your Spirit

"There's nothing more nourishing to the spirit than doing what you feel called to do." -Megan Shull

Any living object which is nourished reflects the appropriateness of that nourishment through changes, usually growth of some kind. The spirit is no exception. To appreciate the effectiveness of the nourishment provided to your spirit we will need to discuss the emotional Positioning system (EPS). Briefly we have learnt that when our bodies are appropriately nourished, we have a change in our physical bodies and it's function. The effect of both over and under nourishment of our bodies is readily visible in our environment. Similarly, the appropriateness of the nourishment of our mindset leads to changes in the way we think and increases our scope and belief in what is possible. We see the effect of this among the dreamers and their accomplishments in our environment. Nourishment of our spirit leads to a change in our emotional states, be it leading to happiness or it's inverse, sadness. Though we may not yet appreciate how this change in emotional states came by, we have doubtlessly seen it in action among our peers and those who cross our paths. I believe that to gain a clear understanding of how nourishment of our spirit impacts our emotional state we must visit the EPS on which we will clarify how nourishment of any type positive or negative impacts our spirit by leading to changes in our emotional states.

Your spirit is waiting to offer you a bounty of goodness.

Caring for your spirit is essential when looking to elevate your life. If you nourish your spirit appropriately it will reward you, no doubt! This is part of its design.

What is nourishment for your spirit, and how can it be provided?

Nourishing your spirit involves taking care of your emotions. As mentioned before the emotional component of your thoughts is the nourishment for your spirit and in turn helps your spirit to be free to give back to you. Like a Global Positioning System (GPS) that you may use when driving or travelling, which gives you the guidance to get to your desired destination, you have an internal navigation system that you are born with which helps guide you through emotional states to the preferred emotional state of your spirit. It is the Emotional Positioning System (EPS) which is inherently a part of you and reflects the status of your spirit. You can think of your EPS as a co-pilot in your emotional life. Just as a GPS system navigates you towards your destination from point A to B, your EPS navigates you towards emotions that will lead to greater joy and abundance in your life.

The Emotional Positioning System (EPS)

The Emotional Positioning System is composed of a variety of levels of emotions listed from number 1 to 21. The various emotional levels which comprise the EPS are listed below. Your spirit is nourished as your emotions move closer towards level 1. (So, it is ideal that you remain on the emotional trajectory going towards level #1.)

1. Joy/Knowledge/Empowerment/Freedom/Love/Appreciation
2. Passion
3. Enthusiasm/Eagerness/Happiness
4. Positive Expectation/Belief
5. Optimism
6. Helpfulness
7. Contentment
8. Boredom
9. Pessimism
10. Frustration/Irritation/Impatience
11. Overwhelm
12. Disappointment
13. Doubt
14. Worry
15. Blame
16. Discouragement
17. Anger/Revenge
18. Hatred/Rage

19. Jealousy

20. Insecurity/Guilt/Unworthiness

21. Fear/Grief/Depression/Despair/Powerlessness/Stress

Note that as you get closer to the top of the list you encounter happier emotions. As you go down the list the emotions continue to become less desirable. You want to try to avoid the less desirable emotions. When nourishing your spirit, you can track the appropriateness of the nourishment with your EGS/EPS. The more appropriate the nourishment, the better your emotional state as the movement up your EGS/EPS heads towards level one. You can track in which direction you are going, because as you move in the direction of level one, you feel happier and have a greater sense of joy because you are moving towards your ideal emotional state to welcome wonderful things into your life. What creates this movement from one emotion to the next is your thoughts. Not only do your thoughts establish your belief system and feed your mindset; they also carry an emotional content which directs the emotional guidance system and nourishes the spirit. Your thoughts function as fuel that drives you along the EGS/EPS. In the teachings of Abraham-Hicks this fuel creates a vibrational energy which feeds the spirit and brings it in better alignment with your purpose. The energy created helps move you along this emotional guidance system (EGS/EPS) towards your desired goal.

You must be prepared to show gratitude for your gifts.

Through your expression of gratitude, you encourage your spirit to give increasingly. When you are willing to remain open to the possibility that there is more to you than just your body and your thoughts, your spirit will work synergistically with these two components to create a state of balance and harmony and provide to you that which you requested. When you can find this balance, you will truly set yourself up for a complete revival of self, adding years to your life and life to your years.

It brings us back to the idea of what you can conceive and believe, you can achieve. Your EGS/EPS will be the perfect guide to your emotional state and indicate the suitability of the nourishment for your spirit. The more adequately you nourish your spirit with positivity and encouraging emotional plaudits, the closer you will be to the higher levels of the EGS/EPS and, in return, more in line with achieving your goals. Please be prepared to show your appreciation by expressing gratitude for your gifts. Let us look at an example of how the EGS works in your life.

Let us suppose you wanted to make more money. As we now know, the Universe has an abundance, and you must be willing to receive that for which you asked. But what if your belief is that there are no more jobs available that will pay more than you currently earn? This brings you into a vibrational state that is not in line with receiving more money into your life. There is no belief more money is available to you, so you are blocking receipt of more money. You are not prepared to receive that which you ask for, so your vibrations would not be coordinated, and you would drop to a lower level on the

EGS/EPS. In examining your emotional state, you are in DOUBT, #13 on the EGS/EPS. Now, what if you moved your emotional state into DISAPPOINTMENT because you realize that you have not really put in the effort to investigate all possibilities for finding new work. It may still feel negative, but in fact it has brought you up to #12 on EGS/EPS. So, you have actually improved your vibrational state, and nourishment of your spirit. #11 OVERWHELM may then come into play by spending time looking for a new job. All these small tweaks in your belief system will continue to effectively nourish your spirit and move you into a more compatible vibration guiding you in the appropriate direction up your EGS. Your emotions will improve, and your spirit will feel more nourished. Keeping in mind the adage, "By the yard it's hard, by the inch it's a cinch!" can really help you appreciate the relationship between your spirit and your emotions. Rarely will you find that you suddenly skip a bunch of emotions and find yourself at an elevated level along the EGS. It is generally small steps in the right direction.

Let us pause to temporarily look at those two emotional states, **(a) DOUBT** and (b) **DISAPPOINTMENT**.

Doubt you will realize has a crippling effect on your emotions, there is a lack of belief and hence a lack of drive because you do not believe that there is better. You then succumb to your doubts and hence belief that there is nothing better or that it is not achievable. On closer assessment, this is almost identical to the thought process of a person with a fixed mindset. He doubts that there is anything better so (s)he remains in his/her comfort zone. In fact, if we look at the emotions 13 to 21 on the EGS, they seem to be more commonly found in persons with a fixed mind set.

The emotion of disappointment reflects the emotional state of someone who has begun the process of reflection. (S) He has started to become a participant in his/her own existence. There is an attempt to question what has been happening to you and as you reflect an emotion of disappointment sweeps over you as you begin to realize more could have been done. This quasi self-assessment extends to level 8 on the EGS, the emotional state of boredom. The various emotional states from level 12 to level 8 reflect a mindset in transition between a fixed mindset and a growth mindset. The other levels up to level 1 are more commonly associated with a growth mind set. Again, reflecting on the interconnectedness between the mindset and the spirit, these two together will encourage the physical structure, your body to act. This provides further evidence that all three compartments of the triune clearly work synergistically to reflect the person you are.

This is where having faith can be of comfort. Appropriate nourishment to your spirit will undoubtedly help you climb higher in your EGS/EPS. However, you must start from a place of belief. If we define faith as the substance of things hoped for, the evidence of things not seen, we can more clearly see how faith fits into the functioning of the EGS.

Faith helps because there may be no physical evidence of your desires for a long time. You must stay strong and remember that "if you believe it, you can achieve it" you must also bring yourself into a state of *feeling* like you already are living or experiencing that for which you ask.... The emotional nourishment of the spirit. If we refer to the previous example, you must feel like you are already making more money before you see evidence of it. This is such an important final piece to nourish the spirit. It may really stretch you mentally especially if you are new to the concept of nourishing the spirit (an integral aspect to understanding the BMS Ecosystem.) But you must have faith and trust (believe) that your efforts in raising your vibrational energy will not be for naught.

Reflection:

If I think of something that is happening right now in my life or a goal that I am consciously working on, can I pinpoint where I am on my EGS/EPS?

In this instance, how can I move up the EGS/EPS?

Are there examples that I can use to flush out for myself?

Can I reflect on moments in my life where I have felt each emotion on the EGS/EPS?

Can I relate each emotion to the one above and understand how my vibrations can take me to a higher emotional state?

_____

_____

_____

_____

_____

_____

_____

_____

_____

_____

_____

_____

_____

_____

I hope you are feeling as excited as I was when I first learned about my EGS/EPS. It is an eye opening and inspiring way of ensuring appropriate alignment with the components of the self. While it may take internal readjustments, learning how your emotions and vibrational states work together to nourish your spirit is essential in the process of your revival.

Levels 1 to 3 at the top of the EGS/EPS are the emotions of Joy, Knowledge, Empowerment, Freedom, Love, Appreciation; Passion, Enthusiasm, Eagerness and Happiness compare this with the stated fruits of the spirit; Love, Joy, Peace, Patience, Kindness, goodness, faithfulness, gentleness, and self-control. These Levels seem in capsule form to be an embodiment of the fruits of the spirit. Let us look more closely at one such emotion, **happiness**.

<u>Happiness</u>

Most experts on the science of happiness agree that the term does not refer to fleeting sensations of joy or pleasure. Being happy does not mean that you feel great all the time, nor does it mean that you are always in a good mood. Research suggests that people who experience the greatest overall well-being are not specifically susceptible to intense emotional highs, this is preferred, because such emotional highs are usually accompanied by intense lows. Life on an emotional plateau is more rewarding than life on an emotional roller coaster. Further, feeling good all the time is not attainable.

Science is clear that happiness is not about material possessions. Happiness is related to having a sense of overall satisfaction with life. It is a sense of fulfilment combined with an overall feeling of well-being that you experience daily. This does not mean that a happy person will not have to deal with sadness, anger, or despair, but they know that these feelings are fleeting, they did not come to stay and yes, they will pass. You need to learn how to tolerate and overcome them.

Dr. Seligman, the father of the positive psychology movement, wrote that happiness is only one component of a sense of overall well-being. Well-being to him is composed of five components:

1. Positive emotion – this encompasses all positive feelings e.g. Joy, comfort, and pleasure.

2. Engagement – this relates to the depth to which you absorb the subject.

3. Positive Relationships – relationships with whom you can share your highs and lows.

4. Meaning – relates to the sense of belonging or serving something greater than oneself.

5. Accomplishment – associated with the process in acquiring as opposed to the acquisition.

Happiness and well-being are not goals per se; they are a journey. They are not a fixed acquisition, more the process one goes through to acquire the object. Happiness therefore becomes an ongoing process. There is good evidence that optimism and happiness coexist and both lead to healthier, more successful, and more fulfilling lives.

We must recognize that it takes effort to improve our emotional lives, and that the effort does pay off. Now that we have that piece of the puzzle in place, let us move on to examining the environments in which your spirit will remain nourished and therefore flourish!

Chapter 12: The Best Environment to Nurture Your spirit

"The best way to cheer yourself up is to try to cheer somebody else up." Mark Twain

In attempting to obtain the best and safest environment in which to nurture your spirit, you will doubtlessly meet negative people along your path. To ensure that your spirit is appropriately nourished, let us explore ways in which you can deal with the negative ones we encounter along the highway of life.

__Negative People__

Negative people seem talented in bringing down any progress which you have made, be it towards your happiness and well-being or almost any other sphere of your life. It is therefore palpably important to be capable of addressing these people to sustain your happiness and well-being and so add years to your life and life to your years.

Step 1: Cultivate boundaries, never seek advice from a negative person. Interestingly, these people are always willing and ready to offer advice, even if that advice is unsolicited. Be prepared to establish boundaries, even if you may be unfamiliar with the individual offering the advice, do a quick assessment of where that person is in life and determine if that is where you see yourself going, if the answer is no, then discard the advice without a second thought.

Step 2: Accept them for who they are and make an informed decision about how you want or need them in your life. You need to determine the significance of these people in your life, what do they contribute to your growth, your mindset, or your person. You may realize that they make a light contribution to your mood or your exercise program and as such you only engage them in these activities, maybe sharing a joke or maybe go to the gym with them but outside of those entities you do not consider them as 'your friends' with whom you spend quality time or with whom you engage in meaningful discussions. In other words, you have categories of friendships or friends for occasions. For example, as a medical doctor, I have been amazed by the offerings of folks. I met a fraudster masquerading as a project manager who offered to train me to speak publicly at a cost. Our paths quickly changed direction with mine going in the opposite direction from his. One must therefore be cautious of those who are making offers that they cannot deliver.

Step 3: Avoid trying to win one against a negative person. For example, a person complaining about the behavior of her teenage son, don't try to outdo her by claiming that your own son has a drug issue. If you find yourself doing this, try to nip it before it starts to fester.

Step 4: Be an adult. If a negative person needs support or reassurance give it to them, if they need to be right let them be right. Try to avoid arguments with a negative person because they will win every time, bringing you down to their level.

Step 5: Recognize and know that it is all right to walk away from a negative person. Be prepared to do so even if they are family members, though this may be initially difficult, but by gradually creating distance between yourself and that person you may achieve the desired goal.

Step 6: If you are the boss and an employee is always negative, recognize that this attitude could have an impact on the work environment, affecting productivity and employee morale. Be prepared to address this even if it means terminating the employee. As is frequently said, one bad apple spoils the whole lot, don't allow one negative person to destroy your business. Remember the environment can influence your mindset and create difficulty in nurturing your growth.

Step 7: You are all about creating positivity, so your effort should be focused on building a network of positive people which will be an ideal environment for nourishing your spirit.

You need to be a happy human being! As we have discussed in the previous chapter your emotions indicate if your spirit is being adequately nourished. Your spirit will also guide you towards environments that will provide the best nourishment and prevent you from falling prey to negative emotions. The adage "Birds of a feather flock together" is applicable here. Abraham-Hicks teaches us, your spirit will seek out elements which have the same vibration as your own. You may not realize it, but you have already experienced this in one way or another.

Have you ever been in the company of someone, and you just do not jive with them, even though you cannot find anything wrong with them per se? Or you have been at a gathering or event and have the desire to leave even though there really is nothing wrong. Upon entering you felt good and were looking forward to enjoying yourself but shortly after you stepped into the room something did not feel right and you wanted to leave? This is the reaction of your spirit meeting energetic vibrations that do not align. Your spirit wants to be in the company of people whose spirit is in harmony with your own because it facilitates your happiness! Be mindful that as you continue to revive yourself, you may find your spirit not vibrating on the same plane as other people who have usually felt close to you. If your vibrational alignment shifts, so may your desire to be around particular people. Be aware of this phenomenon.

Natural Laws and the Law of Attraction

Natural laws are objective and universal and exist independently outside of general human understanding and society at large. Just as morality (what we view as right and wrong) applies to everyone, so do the natural laws. The natural laws are written about by scholars. There is one law, in particular, that is directly associated with the creation of the appropriate environment that ensures that your vibrations are in alignment. When your vibrations are synchronized, it facilitates appropriate movement along the EGS/EPS. Your spirit is then nourished, and your emotions may reach an appropriate level on the EGS, that is moving towards level 1. The natural law is The Law of Attraction.

A simple workable definition for the law of attraction is found in Abraham-Hicks's teachings as "that which is like unto itself is drawn." In other words, like attracts like, and positive or negative thoughts may bring positive or negative experiences into your life. This may seem to have manifested itself repeatedly in our lives, and we have accepted it for what it is. But is it true? Does it work on occasions but not on others? Could there be another component to this law to make it true in your life?

The law as stated is an oversimplification and lacks a key element before it can be a natural law which works every time. The law is not as simple as stated. There is a **bridge** needed to attract like to like. Think of two identical pieces of metal lying side by side. They are the same, yet they exist as two separate items. But if one piece of metal is magnetized? Then the pieces of metal would be magnetically attracted to each other and stick together. This magnetization is the bridge attracting like to like. You may quickly and rightfully argue that this phenomenon only occurs with metallic substances and magnetized substances. Would it still apply to pieces of lumber? Of course, We cannot magnetize lumber, but we can get lumber sticking to each other by applying a bridge, be it glue, nails or some other bridging entity. The message here is simply to get like to stick together or even attract each other, there is need for a bridge. Since attraction is not always evident, consideration to renaming the law of attraction to the law of bridging is appropriate. The law of attraction is a catchier name and is unlikely to change but as stated it can be misleading. In your own life, this sort of bridging energy is necessary when working with and applying the Law of Attraction. In our human form, this magnetization is our

FOCUS.

The required level of focus is reflected in a common saying by Les Brown who claims that if you want something bad enough you will go out and fight for it, you will work day and night for it, you will give up your time, your peace and sleep for it, If all that you dream and scheme is about it....with the help of God you will get it. This reflects intense focus what is described as the **FLOW** by Psychologist Dr Mihaly Csikszentmihalyi, one of the founders of the positive psychology movement. Dr Csikszentmihalyi describes six key features of the **FLOW**:

1. It involves intense focused concentration on the present moment.

2. Causes action and awareness to merge.

3. There is a loss of self – consciousness, this may lead to a temporary loss of sensations such as hunger and pain.

4. There is a keen sense of personal control.

5. You lose track of time.

6. The activity is pleasurable or rewarding, regardless of the potential goal or outcome.

Flow he contends can occur because of both professional and leisure activities. There is increasing evidence that people who are routinely able to attain a state of **FLOW** are happier overall.

People have attempted to unravel this puzzle, and several have hinted at the failure of this supposedly natural law, since it occasionally fails to withstand scrutiny. We have mentioned the saying "what you conceive and believe, you can achieve." Simply conceiving is not sufficient, the element of belief becomes a necessary ingredient, the "magnetizer" if you will. The depth of our belief determines our focus and activates the Law of attraction. Therefore, the law of attraction fails to exist without the appropriate magnetization or focus. The focus of your thoughts will magnetize and attract other similar (like) thoughts and feelings. These magnetized aspects will also attract to you anything that is on the same vibration. Please be mindful that this applies to thoughts good or bad. You must be aware of how you are feeling and what thoughts are bringing you into these emotional states, as you will attract what you are feeling and thinking based on the degree of energy or focus you place on the feeling or thoughts. You want to ensure your focus is appropriate so that it will serve you, attracting that which you desire!

Interestingly the role of magnetization is not new and has long been practiced in the Christian community. Faith in the bible is the assurance of things hoped for, the evidence of things not seen. As the bible says repeatedly, ask and it shall be given. However, it is the faith that one has which magnetizes this "request" and the gifts from God. This is stated most clearly in the new living translation bible in Mathews chapter 21 and verse 22; you can pray for anything, and if you have faith, you will receive it. Prayer demonstrates faith. Praying is the act of requesting but your faith brings into focus that for which you ask. Evidence of the law of attraction and focus at work can be

138

seen in this scenario.

Case in point, you have just bought a new car, and suddenly you start seeing more cars on the road like the one you just bought. Do you believe that it is because of the Law of Attraction that your new car simply attracts these other cars which were hardly noticeable before you purchased your new car? Is it that since you bought your new car everybody has now bought and is driving the very same vehicle that you bought? Surely, you will agree that is not a rational way to think about it. But a more reasonable lens to see this through is that since your focus has now changed, you are now noticing cars like yours as you drive. The question then becomes how do you create the bridge from thought to reality in your own life?

Reflection:

Can I remember a time where the company I was in made me feel "off" or uneasy?

How did it make me feel when I did not leave?

What are my thoughts on the Law of Attraction?

Can I think of something right now that I have been trying to manifest but have not been putting in the work or focus required to magnetize it and attract it to me?

_____

_____

_____

_____

_____

_____

This aspect of your spirit continues to be a fascinating and rich part of your revival. It can all seem so simple and yet so complicated. Now that you understand the law of attraction and how through your own focus, you can make it a working part of your life, let us go back to discussing your Emotional Guidance System/Emotional positioning system (EGS/EPS). Together with your comprehension of the law of attraction and your EGS/EPS, we can begin exploring how things outside of yourself may impact your spirit. Remember that all these aspects are working closely together to revive your spirit and must be in place to bring more years to your life and life to your years.

Chapter 13: Factors that Impact our Spirit

"We have nothing to fear but fear itself." - *Franklin D. Roosevelt*

As you can see, your spirit wants to keep you comfortable and happy in your life. Your spirit wants to support you and be an advocate for you in times of need. It is beautifully intertwined with your emotions. Your emotions can function as an indicator of the state of your spirit and if you are in line with the higher vibrations of your potential.

If something or someone impacts you emotionally, you know your spirit is going to be affected. This may look like unsolicited advice, inappropriate comments, a sudden loss, or a yearning for the beauty of the forest, etc. Without warning these are things that may trigger your emotions. Your spirit is impacted in many ways. To ensure you have control and work with this to your advantage, let us review your Emotional Guidance System (EGS/EPS). Let us further explore how you can empower yourself in aiding your spirit to be safeguarded from circumstances that may impact you.

Revisiting the Emotional Guidance System (EGS/EPS)

A quick reminder that your EGS/EPS has two terminals and a plethora of emotions in between. You can determine where you are and in which direction your emotions are headed (higher or lower vibrational state) based on movements and changes in your emotions.

141

As previously compared, our EGS is like an internal GPS.

GPS systems only work because of the input of external factors such as traffic, road closures etc. A GPS system collects data from multiple external sources so that it may guide you to your destination as quickly and efficiently as possible. Similarly, the emotions that your EGS/EPS is founded on will undoubtedly be impacted by outside sources, therefore directing your EGS direction. You are either heading to bright and joyful emotions or continuing down through negative emotions. In both the GPS and EGS systems, a pilot is needed. That is, **you**. You have the power within you to ensure your EGS is steered in the right direction.

When external factors begin affecting your emotions, it is necessary to understand when you are engaging with your belief system or just fleeting thoughts that are popping up occasionally. I like to frame these as chronic thoughts and acute thoughts. Chronic thoughts are ones that you are constantly thinking or that are long standing, and thus create your belief systems. While your acute thoughts are ones that just seem to pop up and leave as quickly as they arrive. The impact of external factors on our thoughts will always be determined by you. For you to have a clear understanding of this and how it impacts you, let's take a look at a situation where the chronic and acute thought systems come into play. Remember, your attention to the matter enhances your focus and therefore magnetizes your goals and desires.

The EGS/EPS at Work

Let us dive into a relatable example of how your thoughts and EGS can work for you or against you. The key is you must be willing to work with managing your belief system.

Lisa is morbidly obese and has been trying to lose weight for some time. She has tried at least three different weight loss programs but with no success. Because of these failures Lisa begins harboring negative thoughts that diets do not work and will begin to develop a belief system around diets. Lisa's friend introduces her to a new diet that she has been trying for 3 months with noticeable plausible results. After some coercing from her friend, Lisa decides to try this new diet plan even though she now holds a strong belief that diets don't work, and she does not expect to be successful.

Lisa's chronic thoughts and emotions around diets have created a belief that this diet will not work. So how is it to be expected that this diet will offer results when Lisa is living in a vibration of believing that it will not? Lisa's thoughts ("diets don't work") and her desires ("I want to lose weight") do not match up! If they do not match up, based on what we know with how the EGS/EPS works and how the Law of Attraction can be activated through magnetization, of course she will continue to fail. The magnetization in this case is based on Lisa's chronic thoughts, her focus, that diets do not work. It is her belief system and since she believes that diets do not work, her focus will draw thoughts and behaviors to her magnetized belief system ensuring that this diet plan will not work.

Even Lisa's actions will remain in line with her beliefs of the diet not working. If portion control is in question, she is much more likely to not adhere to her diet's guidelines. To her, it is foolish to make the sacrifice by controlling her portion sizes when she knows diets do not work. Since her focus is that diets do not work, she will attract thoughts and behaviors which will ensure that this diet will also fail – the law of attraction in action. When she checks her weight and has gained weight because of not following her diet guidelines, she will then have demonstrated the workings of the law of attraction and find herself falling further down her EGS/EPS. In this example, Lisa has asked the Universe to facilitate her weight loss (acute thoughts) but because her acute thoughts were not synchronous with her belief system ("diets don't work," chronic thoughts,) she was not prepared to receive her gift of weight management.

This is an example demonstrating that to obtain that for which you seek, your belief system and acute thoughts <u>must</u> be in alignment. You must be prepared to receive that for which you asked. Your attention to things which activate opposing vibrations to your desires will lead to a failure in your receiving your desire. Your focus and the resultant magnetization will shift your vibrations in the direction of your focus, in this example, diets don't work. The result is the fulfillment of your belief, your focus, diets do not work. The vibrations of your chronic thought opposes the vibrations of your acute thoughts with the result that your chronic thoughts vibrations overrides the acute thoughts leading to your failure in acquiring that which you requested, which would be a product of your acute thoughts. Your acute thoughts are that which you requested and your chronic thoughts form your belief system. The interplay between your acute and chronic thoughts will prevent you from acquiring what you desire in life unless they are in alignment. Take immediate responsibility for what you are and are not bringing into your world. Begin examining different areas of your life and see if you have some goals in play that do not seem to be getting you anywhere.

Dig deep and notice if you have beliefs in different areas that are preventing you from moving forward and moving up in your EGS towards more joy and happiness. You must remove the discord between your desire (acute thoughts) and your belief (chronic thoughts). As we have mentioned, once you have recognized that your chronic and acute thoughts may be playing against each other, it is then time to clarify what you need and hence enhance your focus, which may bring you into the '**FLOW**'; deep focus and concentration thus facilitating your movement ahead. Remove distractions and ensure that your desire (acute thoughts) is in line with your goal (chronic thoughts). The Universe will have no choice but to activate the law of attraction, to support your chronic thoughts and deliver your goal to you.

Reflection:

When have my chronic thoughts (or belief system) taken me further away from a goal I desire?

Can I see a direct correlation in my life when my acute thoughts and chronic thoughts were not in alignment and therefore prevented me from achieving my goal?

Reflect on a time in your life when you asked the universe for something, for example money to pay your utility bill. You have no idea where the money is coming from, but you are focused on acquiring the money. Has the universe delivered the money to you?

_____

_____

_____

_____

_____

_____

_____

_____

Belief and Faith

In our example with Lisa, if she embarked on the new weight loss plan harboring thoughts such as "I know this works and I have seen great results in my friend", she would be starting out from a great place because her chronic thoughts would be strong and she would be focused on the positive. She would start believing that since it worked for her friend, she was determined to make it work for her. Lisa is focused. She wants to bring herself in line with her goal. She would heighten her focus, leading to magnetization and activation of the law of attraction which would attract factors which when employed by Lisa would allow her to obtain her goal. She will focus on how the program will work if she follows it and this will magnetize more positive thoughts to her. Lisa would then begin seeing the fruits of her effort which would then cause her to feel better about herself and inspire her to stay on a disciplined track with the new diet. Her emotions would shift causing her to get higher on the EGS and closer towards reaping the fruits of her spirit.

This is how faith works in activating the law of attraction. What you think of will attract its vibration towards you. You must trust that this is the case. You must believe that even though you cannot see it now, you will achieve it. Faith is that focus necessary to magnetize your desire so that you can achieve your goal. You have faith in the process, and you have faith in the future outcome. As you continue to climb higher on your own EGS, you feel a sense of relief and a willingness to keep believing.

Reflection:

Can I think of an example where I honestly believed in something and was able to climb higher on my EGS and in turn attract what I wanted towards me?

How does it make me feel to have faith and be willing to keep trying?

What stands in the way of my greatness?

_____

_____

_____

_____

_____

_____

_____

_____

When trying to create change in your life, your role is to constantly reach for a feeling of improvement. You can actively cultivate tools to facilitate your positivity, thereby minimizing the effects of negativity on your spirit. Interestingly, when you relax, your brain waves, muscles, heart rate, even breathing and all your bodily processes are in a calm state but these change and become more excitable as you become agitated. Experts have advised that through a sort of biofeedback mechanism you should attempt to use information on the biological processes in your body to help train yourself into a positive mental and physical state.

This may involve focusing on the biological process of your

own breathing and may facilitate a sort of feedback loop leading to a calmer you. Journaling may allow for the development of new skills and practices which promote happiness and well-being. Dr Siegel contends that the act of writing down our stories activates the narrator's function in our minds allowing us to process the event fully and thereby prevent it from provoking current unexpected physical and emotional responses. Journaling is a way of making sense of our past and allowing us to overcome trauma and adversity and finally, through meditation we can train our brain to go to a peaceful, happy, or relaxed state and thereby stave off an agitated state.

By employing these three entities or combinations of these entities, we can develop skills to allow us to cope with the difficulties of daily life and allow us to develop happiness and a sense of well-being.

Coping Mechanisms

The American poet, Lanston Hughes, reminds us in his poem *Mother to Son,* that "...life is no crystal stair, there are tacks in it, splinters, board torn up and places with no carpets on the floor, bare, ... "

Martin Luther King Jr chided us that it is only when it is dark enough can we see the stars. So, we know that despite our efforts, there will be challenges, and we will need to find coping mechanisms if we are to keep going forward. It is easy to stay positive and emotionally happy when times are good but when things go wrong our coping strategies are tested. It is in this scenario that familiarity with and understanding of the BMS Ecosystem and its principles rises to the fore and liberates you from the clutches of the malaise.

Our sense of purpose and our social connections can prove dramatically helpful to our physical well-being. It is true we mentioned in section one the benefits of healthy eating, exercising, temperance, sunlight, water, rest, and air. These are essential elements in maintaining a healthy physical body, but it takes more to be healthy. Too often we pay reduced attention to our emotional health, which is just as important as our physical health, if we are to enjoy the addition of years to our life and life to our years. As reflected on the EGS, if our emotional health is cared for, we can enjoy the fruits of the spirit with its remarkable attributes.

The EGS will indicate to us the status of our emotional health. If our emotional state is not at the upper levels often, then we need to address this; otherwise, our physical health suffers. As indicated above, the upper levels of the EGS are synonymous with a positive or growth mind set. The literature is replete with the benefits to your physical, mental, and spiritual health and the contribution this makes to adding years to your life and life to your years when you develop a positive mindset and hence keep your emotions within the upper levels of your EGS.

Try to determine why you are in an unsatisfactory emotional state. Is there a lack of meaning in your day-to-day life or is your circle of socialization too small, lacks variety or interest? If so, try new activities. This will allow you to establish new contacts, keep active and generate interest in your life. Reach out to classmates, hear their stories,

reminisce on school days, have a laugh, start a social media group....
Being a part of a community has immeasurable benefits, not least of
all Catharsis.

If the unsatisfactory emotional state is the result of
interpersonal conflicts, set boundaries. Avoid spending time with the
people with whom there is a conflict. Alternatively, improving your
communication with that individual by becoming more empathetic and
a more active listener could help to reduce the conflict which would
be mutually beneficial.

If the cause of your unsatisfactory emotional state is because
of a change in your life, be it major physical injury, a divorce or even
the death of a family member, cognitive flexibility will help you to
cope. Simply put, it is a way of thinking and seeing things in a unique
way. For example, maybe if you are going through a divorce. Cognitive
flexibility may involve you thinking about the positive benefits of
divorce. In the case of the death of a family member, being able to
reminisce on the good times you have had with that person and the
fact that your life was more fulfilled for having them around will most
definitely help you to cope. Falling back on your signature strengths
(the abilities that contribute to our happiness and well-being and that
come easy to us) will prove to be a useful ally when coping with bad
news.

You will know that you are moving in the right direction by a
drift in your emotions toward level one on the EGS which will lead to
you bearing the fruits of the spirit that you seek. It is always there for

the taking. But as discussed, I urge you to not allow your old beliefs to get in the way. Be prepared to get out of your own way and **BE THANKFUL**. This is about your life now. This is about your revival! You have the power to create a life filled with joy and vitality. I believe in you!

Chapter 14: Bringing It All Together

"Everyone has inside of him a piece of good news. The good news is that you do not know how great you can be! How much you can love! What you can accomplish! And what your potential is!" - Anne Frank

It is evident that you are much more complex than meets the eye. You go way beyond just your physical body, and you are a multilayered and interesting entity. It is up to you to develop the triune, **'you',** in whatever capacity you wish. I must remind you that whichever point of the journey you are on in your life, it is not too late to start from where you are. Willing or not, changes are constantly taking place within you and around you, thus, you have a choice. You can be an active participant and marshal those changes to serve in your revival. Or you can be a passive attendant and simply observe the changes as they happen year after year. The choice is YOURS and yours alone. Do you wish to be a bystander in your life, or an active participant?...

A bystander gives up their ability to choose, either willingly or loses it. Either way, the bystander lacks the control of their destiny, has sacrificed their authority and ability to guide their life to a desired location. When you choose to be a bystander in your life, you become complacent and just accept all that happens to your body, mind, and spirit with each passing year.

An active participant, on the other hand, retains a personal stake in the direction of their journey, creates goals and targets their approach to their desired destiny. They stay aware of how they are growing and developing in their body, mind, and spirit, and remain committed to growing each part of themselves. To simply exist is not their idea of how they want to live their life.

After thoroughly examining the triune of which you are composed, I trust you feel empowered to play a more active role in your revival. You now have the tools to nourish, adapt to appropriate environments, and protect each component of yourself from negative aspects of life that can adversely affect your person. It is now up to you to commit to your revival and add years to your life and life to your years.

Any positive activity you perform has an impact on all components of yourself. A notable example of this is the act of physical exercise. When you exercise you are strengthening the muscular and cardiovascular systems and contributing to your weight management. However, when we move our body, our brain also releases endorphins which improve our mood and give us an emotional "high", affecting both the mind and the spirit. It results in the appropriate movement along our Emotional guidance system. Every action has a reaction, no matter which component of yourself is working. They are all intertwined, and every action counts.

No one tries to run away from things that are good for them. They run full steam ahead into them and embrace the great possibility of living a full and rich life! This is what I wish for you and why I wanted to share this revival process. We are triunes, and we must have all three components of ourselves working in harmony to really reap the rewards of your efforts.

Reflection:

What is the biggest take-away I have personally learned about my body?

My mind?

My Spirit?

What was the biggest "ah-ha!" moment in reading this book?

What is something I can start working on right away to serve my revival?

What is the one thing I would want to share with someone I love?

_____

_____

_____

_____

_____

_____

_____

_____

_____

Final Thoughts...

There is a potency which results when all three elements are aligned which forces the universe to take note and create a healthier and more dynamic life for you. My favorite example of this is my paternal Grandmother. She lived to the grand old age of 115 years! (She was recognized as the eldest woman on earth for years.) What was her secret you may ask? It was not simple luck, or great genetic make-up. She was active and vibrant with unwavering faith. You could see that all parts of her fed each other to create a synergy and vibrancy to her life. In my mind her life bore testimony of a dedication to the revival and adding years to life and life to your years.

Further evidence emerges from this nun's study that gives a broad insight into tools which convey longer and productive lives. In this study, 1,932 Nuns wrote a biochemical sketch of their lives. Based on their sketches, the Nuns were divided into four groups. Nuns whose sketch revealed the most positive and optimistic feeling were in group A. In group D were those whose sketches revealed the least optimism and were the most negative, the other two groups were in between these two extremes. After 85 years, 95% of the Nuns in group A were still living active lives whereas only 34% of the nuns in group D were alive; after 90 years, 54% of the Nuns in Group A were still alive and only 11% of those in group D were alive. That is remarkable, isn't it? Is this the result of luck or good genes? Surely it could be neither because the only thing the nuns in group A had which the nuns in group D did not have is a difference in optimism and positivity. It was their mindset that truly set them apart, and as we have discussed I am sure that because our three components of body, mind and spirit interact, the positivity in their minds most certainly affected the whole of their lives. As we can clearly see, the potent forces of the Universe will take note of your efforts and reward you with years to your life and life to your years.

The value of this phenomenon is explored in the positive psychology movement. This movement has thus far revealed the countless benefits to be had on your longevity, health, and happiness through positive thinking.

My deepest passion and one of my life missions is to share this process of revival with as many people as I can! You *deserve* to live your best life well into your golden years. Imagine being able to see your grandchildren grow into independent adults and allow you to spend quality time with your great grandchildren?... It is possible!

I look forward to connecting more with you in the future. Take diligent care of your body, mind, and spirit, and in turn, enjoy the benefits of living the most vibrant days of your life yet!

Dr. Harris Phillip is available as a guest speaker, for interviews and for seminars, consultations and workshops. Look forward to his future series of seminars and his workshops, "Don't Just Tell Me, SHOW ME." To find out more and to book please check out his website:

www.philburnacademy.com

Do not hesitate to pop him an email if you have any questions or are interested in engaging his services!

Acknowledgements

Certainly, Rome was not built in a day, and so I pause to appreciate all who have in myriad ways helped me to become who I am today. I am acutely aware and believe that all that I am and ever hope to become was not simply born out of my innate characteristic but instead is a product of a multiplicity of influences whom I acknowledge and to whom I say thanks.

On reflection, I genuinely acknowledge and say thanks to everyone who has contributed to my existence to date. Every encounter, every interaction, every challenge, every resistance was but an additional building block in my personal development.

To my informal teachers, my earliest educators, my immediate family, parents and siblings, your efforts at teaching me early the differences between right and wrong and protecting me from myself is a major reason I am here today and so for that I thank you.

From my teachers at all levels of my formal education beginning from my earliest kindergarten days through to elementary school, through to high school, college, and university, you all made a significant contribution to my growth and training and to you I extend my gratitude.

To my various students at high school and university levels in the Caribbean, USA, and the UK. Thanks for your contribution to my education and growth. Each of you in your own distinct and individual way made a definite impact on me and who I have become today. Because of your contributions, I continue to grow year after year not only as a teacher but as a human being.

To my patients, your confidence and trust in me, coupled with the opportunity you gave me to be involved in your care, has served me well and for your unique contributions to my growth, I extend my gratitude.

To my acquaintances and friends, I say thanks for your friendships and interactions over the years. Through various discussions and conversations, you have made an indelible impact on me and continue to leave an imprint on my person.

To my current life coaches and mentors, I am eternally grateful for your continued invaluable contributions. I will continue to strive to ensure that your guidance and training have not been in vain.

As you can see, I have stayed clear from name calling. I have always found that to be divisive and essentially double edged. My aim is to level the platform of individual contribution since everyone with whom I traversed paths has contributed to my growth in some way. I see myself as being carried around on the shoulders of all those with whom I come into contact, and I acknowledge everyone no matter how small or large your impact.

My deepest and heartfelt thanks… everyone.

Biography – Long

Harris E. Phillip, MD has been practicing medicine for more than three decades, with a focus as a consultant Obstetrician and Gynecologist. Harris received a BSc (summa cum laude honors) in Chemistry and a MSc in chemistry, before proceeding to spend a year in the PHD program in Organic Chemistry at Texas A&M University. He also possesses an MBBS degree, Doctor of Medicine (DM) degree and a Master's degree in Law (LLM degree). Harris is a fellow of both the American College of Obstetricians and Gynecologists and the Royal college of Obstetricians and Gynecologists (UK), and he is a former Chairman and Vice-chairman of the junior fellows of the American College of Obstetricians and Gynecologists.

Harris' work is widely published in international medical journals, and he has contributed to an array of print and online educational tools in the medical field. He is currently a reviewer for 11 international journals and helps to determine what is medically acceptable and publishable in those journals. Beyond his own practice, he has also lectured nursing students, nurses, midwifery students, midwives, medical students, as well as junior and senior medical doctors for over 20 years.

His current passion lies in helping you live your best life through understanding that when your body, mind and spirit are all cared for in equal manner, you will truly be able to lead your best life! www.philburnacademy.com

Biography – Short

With more than 30 years as a practicing MD and over 20 years lecturing health care professionals, Dr. Harris Phillip is enthusiastic about you achieving your highest level of health which will ensure that you live your best life. He believes that not only do you have to take care of your body, but also your mind and spirit to achieve a total state of wellbeing that will add years to your life and life to your years! www.philburnacademy.com